PHYSICAL THERAPY SALES BOOK

TO SELL IS HEALTHY

GET THE UNSHAKEABLE CONFIDENCE
TO SELL YOUR PHYSICAL THERAPY SERVICES –
AT TWICE THE PRICE YOU'RE CHARGING NOW

PAUL GOUGH

Paul Gough Publishing

Copyright © 2019 Paul Gough. All rights reserved.

This publication is licensed to the individual reader only. Duplication or distribution by any means, including email, disk, photocopy, and recording, to a person other than the original purchaser, is a violation of international copyright law.

Publisher: Paul Gough, 25 Raby Road, Hartlepool, UK, TS24 8AS

While they have made every effort to verify the information here, neither the author nor the publisher assumes any responsibility for errors in, omissions from or a different interpretation of the subject matter. This information may be subject to varying laws and practices in different areas, states, and countries. The reader assumes all responsibility for the use of the information.

The author and publisher shall in no event be held liable to any party for any damages arising directly or indirectly from any use of this material. Every effort has been made to accurately represent this product and its potential and there is no guarantee that you will earn any money using these techniques.

ISBN: 9781082154645

ALSO BY PAUL GOUGH:

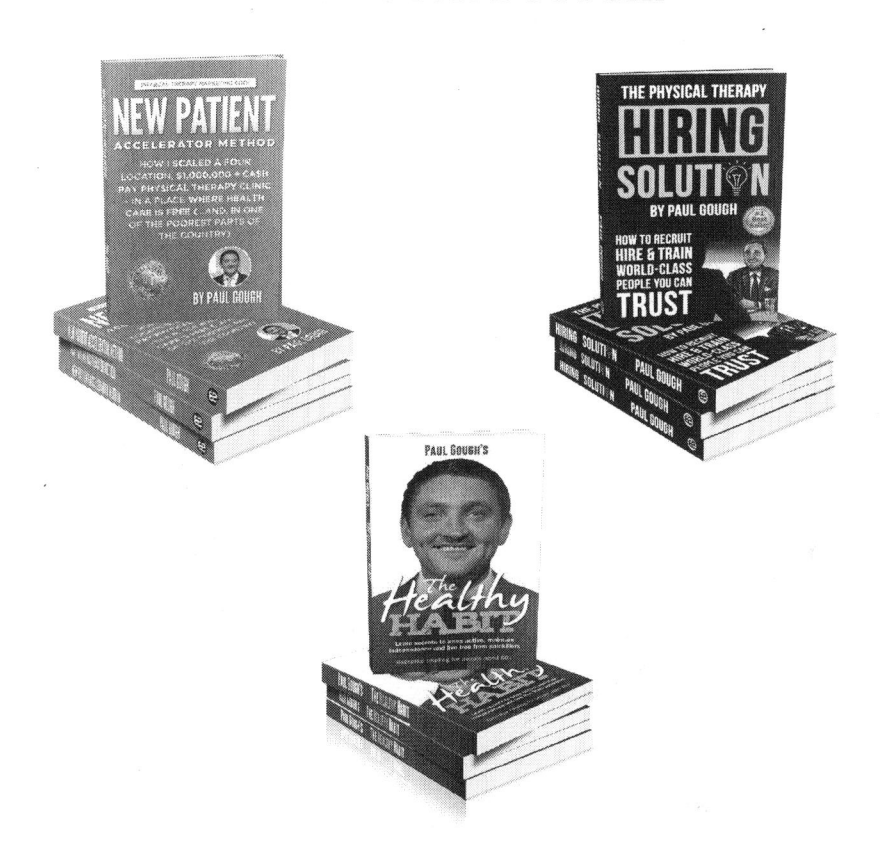

New Patient Accelerator Method:
"How I Scaled a Four Location, $1,000,000 + Cash Pay Physical Therapy Clinic - In a Place Where Health Care Is Free (...And, in One of the Poorest Areas of the Country)"
www.PaulsMarketingBook.com

The Physical Therapy Hiring Solution:
"How to Recruit, Hire and Train World-Class People You Can Trust"
www.PaulsHiringBook.com

The Healthy Habit:
"Learn Secrets To Keep Active, Maintain Independence And Live Free From Painkillers. Essential Reading For People Aged 50+"
www.PaulsHealthyHabit.com

DEDICATION

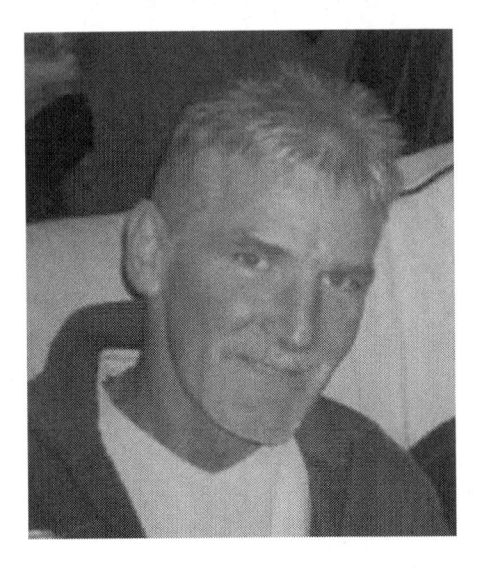

This book is dedicated to the memory of my **Uncle, Liam Gough.**

Liam is/was someone who made me see that confidence and self-belief is a choice; **my choice**. Despite his passing, my Uncle Liam remains hugely influential in my life. To this day, I can still hear his voice in my head telling me to "believe in myself." He told me so many times that in the end, I had no choice but to believe *him*, that believing in *me*, was a good idea.

Most people are searching endlessly for someone to *believe in them*; Liam helped me realize the only person I need to believe in me, *is me* and if I did, anything would be possible. I have no doubt it's one of the reasons you're reading this book today.

That is why, if after reading this book you find yourself with an improved level of confidence and self-belief, then you too can thank my Uncle Liam for that.

I'm sure it would thrill Liam to know that he has directly influenced you and the 10,000's of readers of this book to **believe** that living with **unshakeable confidence** and **self-belief** is not something you have to wait for – it is a choice you're able to exercise starting today.

Uncle Liam, you're the best. I/we are eternally grateful xxx

BEFORE YOU READ THE BOOK DO THIS FIRST...

Just to say thanks for reading this book **I would like to give you a list of the best questions you can ask in ANY sales situation, my check-list to make your front desk phone calls more successful, and a video training to help you stop objections to paying for physical therapy** that are mentioned inside the book – completely FREE!

Go To:
www.paulgough.com/sales-kit
to download it now

Here's What You Will Receive:

- **Instant download PDF** - containing some of the best questions you can ask in any sales situation (incoming calls, drop-offs, cancellations, etc.)

- **Eleven-point checklist** – to make your front desk phone calls more successful

- **Bonus video training** – Paul teaching live from stage on how to stop objections before they even happen

It's All Here:
www.paulgough.com/sales-kit

YOU'LL NEED THIS AS YOU READ THE BOOK...

Go to: www.paulgough.com/sales-kit now
and download your FREE bonus Sales Tool Kit –
it contains many of the resources (and more) that I
mention in the book...

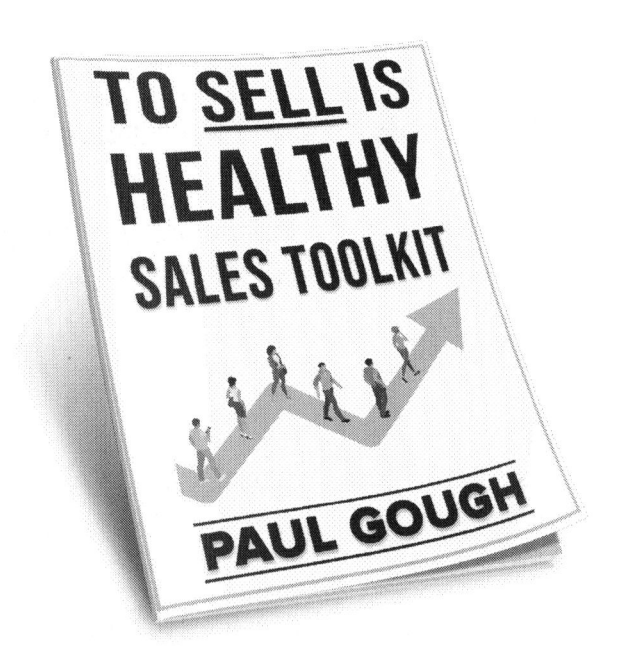

TO SELL IS HEALTHY SALES TOOLKIT

PAUL GOUGH

To get the best out of this book download the
resource PDF now before you start reading:
www.paulgough.com/sales-kit

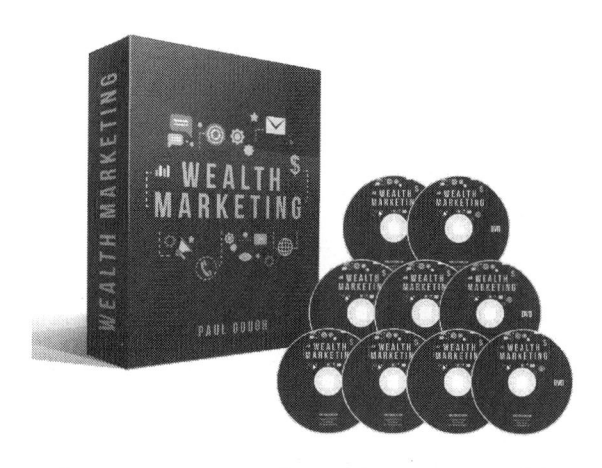

GET YOUR FREE WEALTH MARKETING GIFT FROM PAUL, NOW...

Go to: www.paulgough.com/wealth-gift
To get this instant access 9 DVD video program, NOW.

Claim your $1,997.00 worth of cash patient generating, higher profit making, wealth marketing DVD program, absolutely FREE!

Including a FREE "Test-Drive" of Paul Gough's Cash Club Membership that sends to your clinic $10,000 worth of marketing ideas every 30 days.

Claim your copy now, at
www.paulgough.com/wealth-gift

PRAISE FOR PAUL GOUGH
FROM PHYSICAL THERAPISTS ALL OVER THE WORLD

....

"Before I came across Paul, I didn't know how to handle the cash pay conversation with patients asking about Insurance. What Paul teaches has given me the skills and confidence I needed to handle the money conversation and convert people happy to pay in cash. This new found confidence also allowed me to raise my rates to a big $250 (when I originally planned to raise them to $180!), and I'm hitting my monthly revenue goals."

Stefani Wylie, MPower Physical Therapy Dallas, TX

"Paul has given me (and my team!) the confidence to sell full plans of care, and as a result my cash-pay patients have DOUBLED and keep on coming! Not only do I have a consistent flow of cash-pay, even my insurance patients have started paying in cash and WOM clients keep on coming! Paul has made 'selling' so much easier. So easy that I never really feel like I'm doing it! I was worried about being 'too salesy' when I was trying to sell my services – now it doesn't even feel like I am doing it! Thank you, Paul, you've made my life and business richer."

Hoang Tran, Hands On Physical Therapy, Miami, FL

"Before meeting Paul I lacked the confidence to start my Cash Clinic (in fact, I kept telling myself that opening a cash practice was impossible!) - but really all that was holding me back was the thought that "I had no idea how to sell to a cash-pay market." Paul has showed me step-by-step the things I absolutely must be doing on the phone to convert inquiries, and as a result, asking people to pay in cash is not a problem anymore – in fact, I went back to my new practice and started charging $250 right away!"

Dean Volk, Volk PT, NC and SC

"The biggest struggle I was facing before Paul taught me how to sell, was the ability to convert inquiries and actually get people on schedule. I was painfully uncomfortable discussing cost, and every time the insurance question came up, I would put it off for as long as possible - it scared me! Now I know EXACTLY what to say when the 'dreaded' insurance question comes up with confidence, and I can't remember the last time someone gave me push-back when they heard the cost - I can't believe it, people don't bat an eyelid!"
Danelle Dickson, Performance Plus PT, Washington D.C.

"Prior to discovering what Paul teaches, I was struggling with finding the confidence to sell my services. I was feeling tired, burnt out almost, working part-time at another job just so I could make enough to get by… Paul changed that for me. I was able to understand the psychology behind how people make decisions, how to build trust and learning the importance of follow-up was golden. I've also gone from charging $197 per session to $250, and 6 months later after implementing Paul's strategies I had already made MORE than I had in an entire year."
Tonya Yanok, Yanok PT, Cleveland, Ohio

"How was I able to convert over $6,000 of leads in my first month of business? It's not about me - it's what I learned from Paul Gough! The sales methods Paul shared with me allowed me to gain the social proof to raise my rates before even starting my clinic and gave me the ability to overcome objections - anyone can do this when you apply the principles Paul teaches."
Josh Hall, Hall Physical Therapy, Salt Lake City, Utah

"Before discovering Paul, we most definitely had a sales problem. We've always been a cash practice and had always lived in fear of the dreaded, "Do you take my insurance?" question. Paul has given us a solid strategy and exactly what we needed to answer the insurance question without the phone being slammed down. The results have been stunning."
Tim Gerstmar, Aspire Natural Health, Bothell, WA

CONTENTS

CHAPTER 1
Could Everything You've Ever Been Told About Selling in Health Care Be Wrong? - 7

CHAPTER 2
Seven Reasons Why Physical Therapists Struggle With Selling - 23

CHAPTER 3
Never Forget What You're Actually Selling - 41

CHAPTER 4
Introducing "Effortless Selling" - 47

CHAPTER 5
The Three Most Important Aspects of a Successful Sales Process – 61

CHAPTER 6
Why Patients Really Say "No" – 81

CHAPTER 7

Price is Not the Problem - 95

CHAPTER 8

Common Objections to Physical Therapy - 103

CHAPTER 9

How to Influence with Integrity -

the Five Steps to "Effortless Selling" - 119

CHAPTER 10

Give Yourself a Raise – Effective Today - 131

CHAPTER 11

Get the Complete Sales and Conversion System

For Physical Therapists – 147

"There's no shortage of money and no limit to what people will spend. There's only a lack of imagination"
- Walt Disney

"Talent is being able to sell something you are FEELING."
- Elvis Presley

"Yes, you can get physical therapy cheaper. In fact, I can show you where to get it cheaper from. However, I don't know if it is your experience, but I have never found a company that can offer the best quality and the best service – for the lowest price. May I ask, which are you willing to give up: is it great quality, best service or lowest price?"
- Paul Gough

INTRODUCTION

As you read this book, I want you to keep in mind that I wrote if *for* you. There'll be many times in the book that you'll feel uncomfortable and you might not agree with what I am saying about the often controversial topic of selling in health care.

If at times you do feel uncomfortable, that's okay—that is why I wrote it. Progress *is* uncomfortable and this explains why so many clinic owners don't make that much of it. As I always say, it's very easy to fall asleep on the comfort blanket of the status quo.

In society, in this profession, in general, selling is often discouraged. But is it really all that bad? Is it something that should be frowned upon? Or is it that people get too caught up in the emotional aspect of a bad experience that they've had with a bad sales-person, and assume that all selling is bad?

In this book, I will encourage you to separate "bad" experiences and "bad" salespeople from the very-much-needed process of selling. I'm going to show you a way of selling your services that doesn't feel salesy or leave you wondering if the patient thinks you're being greedy for asking to be paid. More than anything, I'm going to show you how to sell in a manner that is professional, ethical, and done with integrity.

What we're going to cover in this book is a method for selling that puts needs first—the needs of both you and your patients. That is right, we're going to consider *you* for once. It's too easy to think that it's all about the patients when, really, for it to be about the patients, it has to be about the caregivers first (that's you).

I ask you: If the caregivers are not taken care of, then how can the caregivers keep giving care? Most clinic owners are on the rocky road to physical and mental ruin and it's primarily because they can't, won't, dare not, or just flat-out don't know how to charge the prices that would make running a business worthwhile. I'll show you how to do that in this book.

GET YOUR FREE SALES KIT: WWW.PAULGOUGH.COM/SALES-KIT

THE BOTTOM OF THE FOOD CHAIN

For too long, physical therapists have been at the bottom of the food chain, waiting for handouts from doctors and at the mercy of big insurance companies deciding if/when to pay the bills. The best news for physical therapists is that both of those scenarios are not needed anymore. And that isn't fake news.

As far as I'm concerned, doctors can *sell out* their practice any time they like. And as for the insurance companies, they can all go to hell in a handbasket—ideally, as fast as possible, and taking their claims departments to the first available furnace of fire when they get there.

There's an open healthcare market now. And thankfully, patients are waking up to the fact they can use their iPhone to do a Google search and find the solution to their back pain without having to talk to their doctor or insurance.

That's the big opportunity. But the problem that has been created by the big opportunity is that when patients come to you directly or are faced with paying sizable out-of-pocket costs, it's not so easy to get them to buy into your services.

Healthcare costs are on the rise and it's getting harder to get people to part with the money required to pay for the top-class physical therapy that you and I provide. It's not as easy to schedule them as it used to be since many have objections and concerns about cost.

The only way through those objections is to help them to see why, for example, the money you're asking is worth paying, that there is value in paying the fee that you're asking, that there is a legitimate reason they need ten sessions to solve their problem and not the one or two for which they want to pay.

Selling is not always about taking money from people; it's actually more important than that. It's about working with someone to *help them*, to *guide them*, to *support them* and be there to answer their questions so that they can make the absolute best possible decision on what to do about their ailment—however long it takes. If you do that, the money conversation that everyone wants to avoid becomes easy.

I know many physical therapists dread having the money conversation and the irony is it happens because they don't do any real selling. The more you avoid selling, the more uncomfortable the money conversation will be. That's because selling is about building value and showing the person that you're addressing why you're worth paying the price you're asking. If you do it right, the uncomfortable money conversation doesn't exist.

It's only ever uncomfortable in the first place because you don't think they're going to pay. If that's the case, it's because you haven't sold the value of your services. If you haven't done that, you shouldn't expect them to pay. The key is to not shy away from selling, but instead to embrace it.

In this book, I'll show you how you sell in a manner that is ethical, professional, and ensures that the patient receives the outcome that they want. If you do that, you never have to worry about asking for money as they'll *want* to give it to you.

PERMISSION TO MAKE A PROFIT

The thinking that it is wrong to sell in health care is, I believe, the number one thing getting in the way of clinic owners having more success. It is stopping you from making more impact in your community and holds you back from making more money.

And by the way, I firmly believe that the two *can* and *should* go hand in hand. I've said it many times—my clinic is called Paul Gough Physio Rooms, not Mother Teresa's Physio Rooms. We're not a charity and we do exist to make a profit. In fact, the only reason we continue to exist is if we do make a profit. If we don't make a profit, I can't keep the lights on, and I certainly can't pay the people needed to provide a valuable service that changes lives.

Besides, getting the skills required to change someone's life does not come cheap. And when you add on the time, risk, and sacrifice that you make to acquire those skills, you're well within your rights to see a worthwhile return. Not to mention that it usually costs less to see a physical therapist than it does to see a personal trainer or even to get your garage door fixed. Now you can start to see the reasons why you absolutely should be charging more than you are right now.

GET YOUR FREE SALES KIT: WWW.PAULGOUGH.COM/SALES-KIT

To be clear from the get-go, this book is as much about me showing you how to help more people as it is about giving you the **unshakeable confidence** to sell your services at twice the price you are now. Price is a construct. It means something very different to everyone and it's very likely that it's *you* who has the biggest problem with your current prices—not your patients. I'll show you how to price your services in a way that you're comfortable with and at the same time leaves patients happy and feeling as though they received value in paying for it.

What I hope you take from the book is that there is a way to sell that benefits both you and the patient. The dog must wag the tail. Private practice is not a labor of love and never should you feel like you have to keep your prices at the "average" of your town level unless, of course, you think you are average in your town. But I'm sure that's not the case—I suspect you're just a little frightened about losing a patient if you "dare" to charge too much.

I get it. But the goal is surely to serve people who value what you do enough to want to pay for it and, in doing so, make a level of profit that means you can then take better care of yourself and your family. It's called positive capitalism and I'm all for it. What is more, when you make more profit, it also allows you to provide a better level of service that people would be happy to pay for.

Low prices mean Mill-Like service (crappy). I put it to you that people want *more* than Mill-Like service and to get it, they're happy to pay for it. It means you have to charge them appropriately to be able to afford to give it. It is the only way it works. This book is about showing you how to do that and, most of all, to give you the permission to do so.

You're going to discover that what most people think is their real issue with selling actually isn't. It turns out that the real reason you feel more comfortable with giving away discounted treatment, or avoiding the awkward price question altogether, has more to do with the dislike of being *judged* and *rejected* than it does any belief that selling is wrong. As for your issues with money—which aren't your fault—I've been through them too and I'll show you how to get over them in an instant.

I'm also going to show you how to become more comfortable with the silence that ensues after you tell them your price, and how to charge appropriately, free from any guilt or worry that you're taking food off their table or being labeled as greedy for doing so.

GET YOUR FREE SALES KIT: WWW.PAULGOUGH.COM/SALES-KIT

READ WITH AN OPEN MIND

Turn each page and read the book with an open mind. As you do, please know that I'm wanting *you* to be the one who benefits from reading it. I believe that if/when you get the confidence to finally sell your services at a price that reflects the value that you bring, you will be able to impact more lives. Not just your patients, but everyone at home and the people around you. Confidence is infectious.

Right now, the world needs more people with the confidence and resolve to be the absolute best version of themselves. What it doesn't need is another modified or diluted version of a healthcare professional, perpetually worried about what people might think, never quite achieving your full potential because you're always concerned about how you're being judged. In this book I'm going to show you how to stop worrying about being liked and instead focus on being **respected.**

If you're like most physical therapists I meet, I'm pretty sure that if you had a little more confidence, you would be unstoppable in life and in business, and you would go on to achieve more than you ever thought possible. Most importantly, you would live your life without the frustration that comes with trying to please everyone and always hoping that you're not being judged. That's a painful way to live and yet, sadly, it's how most people exist. I hope this book acts a kickstart toward living the kind of life you've always believed possible.

I know at times this is going to feel a little rough and that you will be out of your comfort zone as you do this. But I want you to know that I'm *rooting for you* as you make your way courageously toward telling people that what you do is *going to change their lives*—and that you're going to need to be compensated appropriately for doing so.

What's more, if they don't like it, you're going to love the thrill that comes with telling them how to get an appointment with your much *cheaper* competitor across the street. Best of all, you won't feel anything but joy at doing so as it opens up a spot in your schedule for someone who does value you and what you do; someone who is happy to pay the price you deserve to be paid for the value you bring.

Ready? Let's begin.

GET YOUR FREE SALES KIT: WWW.PAULGOUGH.COM/SALES-KIT

TALK TO ME AS YOU MOVE THROUGH THE BOOK:

LET ME KNOW YOUR THOUGHTS AND COMMENTS OVER ON TWITTER OR INSTAGRAM:

@THEPAULGOUGH // #ASKPG

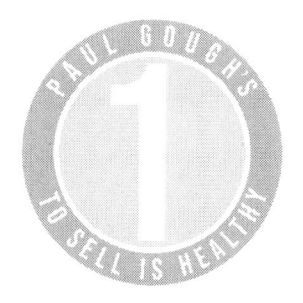

COULD EVERYTHING YOU'VE EVER BEEN TOLD ABOUT SELLING IN HEALTH CARE BE WRONG?

There is a single premise that underlies many of the problems plaguing physical therapists right now. That premise says that it is *wrong* to sell in health care; that it is somehow *unethical* or *beneath* a skilled healthcare professional to sell their patients on the care they need.

It's as if a certificate hanging proudly from the wall makes you exempt from doing something that society has been doing since time began.

For years, we've been made to believe that it's wrong to sell in health care; that it's *not cool* to sell to people if you're a medical professional and, if you do, you're somehow un-professional. Yet, everywhere I look in health care, I see people selling.

I see physical therapists selling themselves to doctors. I see doctors selling out to corporate hospitals. I see companies selling drugs that save lives, as well as tools and equipment that improve medical standards. Not to mention hospitals selling their vacant roles to the best candidates.

The next time you're in the hospital and you're happy with the doctor who cared for you, remember that someone likely sold her on taking the role. After all, and much like your patients, the doctor had many other options for places to work. Someone had to make that role appealing enough for her to want to choose it; someone had to sell it to her. And, because they did, you benefitted from it. The trickledown effect of selling done correctly is that a lot of people benefit. You and I included.

GET YOUR FREE SALES KIT: WWW.PAULGOUGH.COM/SALES-KIT

If the premise is that selling in health care is wrong, then why is it okay in all of these instances? Why is selling accepted and done in almost every other scenario in health care *except* when you're talking to a patient? Why can selling be used to do so much good on one hand and yet on the other, it is demonized as something that no health professional should ever lower their standards to be involved in?

Could it be healthcare's relationship with selling, and how to do it ethically and professionally, is out of date and needs to be cleared up?

Is it because it's falsely assumed that if you're selling, you're trying to get money from people who don't want to give it?

Is it actually nothing to do with selling and everything to do with how selling makes you feel if *you* screw it up?

Or, is that medical professionals are often guilty of hiding behind an expensive qualification and feel a sense of entitlement to patients saying yes—*just* because they're expertly trained?

I believe it is a combination of all of the above and we're going put them all to bed in the pages of this book.

THE BIGGEST PROBLEM GOES WAY BEYOND PAIN

To say that people in our profession have a strong opinion on selling is an understatement—but here's what is wrong with it:

Most have no clue how selling can be used to solve the biggest problem that patients live with that goes way beyond the physical pain they're in.

It's naive to think that the only problem that we need to solve is the one the patient presents with; their back pain or loss of movement in their hip. I propose the real problem is that is they can't decide *what to do* about their back or hip pain.

People have flaws in their ability to decide and those flaws don't go away just because they're in pain. If anything, they get worse when they are in pain. I include myself in this when I say most of us can't even make a decision over what to eat at night, never mind whether to choose a physical therapist over a chiropractor or rest or pills.

And as for asking them to decide over paying cash or using insurance, now you've just tipped them over the edge and back into a world of procrastination. They're back to living with the fear and doubt of making the wrong decision. People can live with pain—but they can't live with the uncertainty that comes with having to take a risk. It's even worse when there are confusing copays or out-of-network expenses involved.

There's not a single human being on Earth that comes pre-programmed with the ability to make good decisions and be comfortable taking risks. That is something that no amount of clinical skills can solve. And yet, to access something like physical therapy, a patient must do both.

The fallacy in physical therapy is that if you have better or more clinical skills, then you don't have to sell. And, in an ideal world, this would be true. The problem is that we live in the *real* world. And in the real world the people we call patients are not as interested in our certificates or Con Ed as we are.

They also still don't really know what a physical therapist even does. "Do you give exercises?" or "Do you treat sports people?" are the typical responses I get when I tell people I am a physical therapist. The list of responses is endless and the only thing consistent is that people aren't really sure what we do.

That is a big problem for us all. If they're unsure it means they're uncertain. If they're uncertain, they're unlikely to decide until someone helps them feel more certain. That's really all we need to aim for in our selling—to help our patients feel more certain about their decision to utilize our physical therapy.

This is why certificates and qualifications are not as important as you wish they were. They're only important when a decision has been reached about which healthcare professional to choose. These things *validate* a decision that has been reached by a patient. But something else entirely is required to help more patients make the decision in the first place.

GET YOUR FREE SALES KIT: WWW.PAULGOUGH.COM/SALES-KIT

That thing is a *certainty in the outcome,* and it is only achieved when they're sold to in a way that is ethical and professional and makes them feel good about what you're about to do. In today's confusing and very crowded healthcare marketplace, there is a need for professionals to recognize that the first place to help people is with making a decision.

Selling is simply a process that, if it is done right, can help people make better decisions faster; it is not always about taking money from people, as is often mistakenly assumed. The two must be separated. When you do that, you can feel more confident in selling.

Change your view that selling is exclusively about taking money from people. Instead, replace it with a view that selling is about helping people feel confident in the money they need to invest in restoring their most prized asset—their health.

Start to see the process known as selling as a way to solve the real problems that all of your patients are living with; that being their inability to decide and their lack of appetite for risk. When you do, you'll help a lot more people.

It's bad for both the profession and the patient to do anything but embrace the fact that selling can be done in a manner that is professional, ethical and *puts the interests of the patients first.* After all, if you shy away from selling someone something they need just because you don't like doing it, whose interest is really coming first?

THE REAL ISSUE WITH ASKING FOR MONEY

Imagine this: you treat a patient and, at the end of the session, for some reason, you don't feel comfortable about asking them for money. You tell them that on this occasion there's no charge. You politely tell them that if they come back next time, then you *might have to charge them* but, on this occasion, you're happy to discount your services to zero.

It's usually done in the name of wanting to help people. But is it *solely* about wanting to help people? Or is there something else going on?

I've spoken to many physical therapists who that tell me that they don't like to sell; that they struggle to ask for payment for their services.

I've even had some who will confess that they're the type who likes to give everything to everyone for free; that it's in their nature to do so. They say it as though it's something to be proud of.

I get it. But I am not sure that this self-labeling is all that accurate.

I *do* agree that they want to help, I'm not debating that for one second. But could it be that what they're really saying is that they don't know how to ask for payment without feeling like they're being judged, or risking being rejected? There's a difference.

This is the real underlying issue with the loathing of selling. It puts you in that awkward position where you can be judged and labeled for being salesy or deemed greedy for charging higher prices. Both of these can make you feel pretty bad about yourself, and once you've experienced either, there's a natural tendency to want to avoid them for good from that point on.

The false assumption about asking for money is that if you take money from people, then you're pulling food from their table. As if getting their back fixed means that they'll have to go without, and you'd be the one responsible for their famine. Of course, all of this is only happening in your head. It's completely made up but it's how many physical therapists feel. Can you relate?

If so, I put it to you that the fear of rejection and the fear of being judged are the root cause of any fear that you're carrying about selling. Having a medical qualification does a great job of putting us on a lofty pedestal—one that you can be knocked down from by being rejected.

It's not so much that you don't want to charge for your services—it's that you don't want to find out that they *don't want to pay for your services.*

When your fees are rejected, it can make you feel inferior. There's no way to neutralize that feeling. The only thing that you can do is try to avoid it altogether. One of the ways you avoid it is to accept the excuse they give you for the reason they can't pay for your services—whatever it is.

If they tell you it's money or time, it's easy to accept because you can pass it off as *their* issue and not one they have with you. In doing so, you instantly mitigate yourself from rejection. Said differently, the reason you're so quick to accept their excuse about a lack of funds is that you never have to find out that the real concern might be *you*.

Instead of considering that there *might* be some other reason for their objection—and challenging that objection ethically—it's easier to accept the price issue and run with a conversation about them having no money (even though they've just told you all about their new Rolls Royce).

IS MONEY EVER THE REAL ISSUE?

Candidly, most of the time it isn't.

It's naively accepted that the only reason that people say no to medical care comes down to money—or a lack of it. But money isn't the true concern for many people. It's the fear of spending it and not being confident in receiving a return. There's a huge difference.

I don't see my patients having an issue spending money on Amazon on stuff they don't need or replacing an iPhone that works perfectly well with a $1,000 upgrade just because a new one came out. Do you?

Truth is, money rarely stops anyone from getting something they *really* want.

If they're not spending money with you, it's because someone didn't do a good enough job of showing them why the figure being quoted is justified. That's what you do in selling. You're selling the value. It's not just about taking money—it's actually about being willing to show why what you have is worth the money you're requesting. It's about showing why they should pay it. There's no profession on earth that is above needing to do this.

Even medical doctors, whether they know it or not, are actively involved in selling their treatment plans to patients with diseases and illnesses. The better they can sell the idea of their suggested treatment, the more people get healthy. The best and most trusted doctors are not just the most clinically skilled, they're also the ones that make you feel *certain* about the otherwise risky surgery that you're about to have. They're the ones selling you on the reasons that you should have the surgery they recommend because they know it'll change your life if you do—or ruin it if you don't.

Selling doesn't mean you're going to be salesy or pushy or even try to persuade someone to do something that they don't want to do. It means you're going to take the time to help them see what you're offering in a different way than they do at the time when they say no.

Selling is simply about helping someone to see something from a different point of view. Selling is about influencing someone with integrity so that you can help them achieve a positive outcome that they couldn't reach without you.

It's why selling is such a magical and profound skill to possess.

Done right, you can help someone to see something that they couldn't two minutes before. For example, you can help someone see how physical therapy is a better alternative to chronic knee pain than more rest and more pills (that so far have not worked).

When what we do is helping them to live more actively, walk further, sleep better, enjoy time with their grandkids, or get back to work to be able to pay their bills—is there any better skill to possess?

The physical therapy profession is constantly telling you that the path to career success is more, more, more, and *even more* clinical skills.

I can be the best physical therapist in my area, but if I can't get people to understand why I need them to book ten sessions with me to be able to ease their nagging lower back pain, then I'm not going make much impact. I'm also not going to make much money.

Only the physical therapy schools that sold you on a $150,000 program (to learn clinical skills) will have you believe that such a thing is possible. You're told throughout physical therapy school that it's wrong to sell in health care; that you won't need to if you're clinically superior. The schools tell you that selling is wrong and they make you feel like it is something dirty and beneath you.

And yet, they're happy to sell *you* on a program costing more than one hundred thousand dollars. It's funny how those lecturers discourage selling, yet if it wasn't for someone *selling their program,* none of them

GET YOUR FREE SALES KIT: WWW.PAULGOUGH.COM/SALES-KIT

would have a job. The world is full of hypocrisy, and it's not just coming from politicians.

MY STRUGGLE WITH SELLING MY SERVICES

Everything I've just mentioned above is what I've been through myself. I spent years worrying over what patients might think of me. And I spent just as long thinking that the reason I couldn't get people to buy into my services was because they didn't have the money to do so.

I started my clinic in a very small town in the northeast region of England (Hartlepool) and it's the type of town where everyone knows everyone. I would go to a bar or restaurant and I was guaranteed to bump into a patient there. Whenever that would happen, I would feel guilty; I stupidly felt as though the person looking at me enjoying my food and wine was thinking that I took money off them to pay for it.

It got so bad that for years I avoided going to restaurants or bars in any of the towns where my clinics were located. On the surface, I would say that I wanted to go somewhere different, but really it was because I didn't want to go somewhere I might be judged.

Thankfully those days are long gone. And not just because I now live in Orlando, Florida, 3,500 miles away. I was well past the fear of being judged phase before I left the UK. The reality is I live in Orlando because I got past that phase.

That's right. As I write this book to you today, I live in Florida, but I remain the proud owner of a successful clinic with over 2,000 visits per month flowing through my four locations in the UK. What's more, we now charge *more* per session than almost every other clinic in all of the UK.

If you're not familiar with my story, I started my clinic—The Paul Gough Physio Rooms—in one of the poorest parts of the UK and scaled it to four sites. We are a mostly "cash pay" clinic, meaning we don't rely upon referrals from doctors or insurance companies to pay the bills. And all of this is happening in a country with a free health care system.

Despite the economic challenges in my area, I'm now able charge more than some of the bigger cities, such as London, where you'd expect people to pay more. For context, think of a clinic in a small town in Louisiana charging more than a swanky clinic in Manhattan.

Gone are the days of worrying over being judged or asking for money for my services. Thankfully, I realized early that most people don't do all that much thinking and, if they do, it's mostly about themselves (myself included). I'm not that special or important that I'll occupy any space in their head regardless of how much money I charge them. These days I care more about the patient not getting the treatment they need than what they think of me. **I focus on being respected not liked.**

This was a huge turning point for me. It was a simple mindset shift that allowed me to go on and build the type of clinic every owner dreams of—a business that generates a significant amount of profit without me having to be there every day. I could never have done that without having the confidence to sell my services at prices that make being in business worthwhile.

But I didn't always have high prices and good profit margins. I started off like most clinic owners with prices that were average, and I suffered regularly from hearing things like "I'll think about it" or "I'll talk to my insurance." As I look back, all of my selling problems started when I left school believing that all my success as a physical therapist hinged on how good of a clinician I was.

And I was a good clinician. I was clinically skilled enough to be able to make it all the way to working at the top level of professional soccer. After five seasons of working with the top soccer players in the UK and learning alongside some of the best doctors in professional sports, I decided to quit my day job and start my own private practice.

I thought that because of my high profile and my high level of clinical skills, I would never have a problem selling my services. But I did. Within weeks of opening up, I was hearing "no" more often than "yes." Even the people who did say "yes" they would rarely see out a full plan of care with me.

I falsely assumed that every objection I ever heard was because of money—or a lack of it. I assumed that it was happening because my patients had the option of free physical therapy paid for by the socialist

GET YOUR FREE SALES KIT: WWW.PAULGOUGH.COM/SALES-KIT

government that offers free medicine to everyone, or that it was because I lived in one of the poorest parts of the country.

I even convinced myself that it was because my town was somehow "different" and folks in my town just don't invest in things like physical therapy. But none of those things were the real truth and thankfully I realized this early.

I believe the reason I went onto grow and scale a four-location clinic that I make money from but don't have to be at every day is because I figured out how to sell to people who are uncertain and skeptical about what we do.

I figured out how to help people overcome the uncertainty they have when choosing things that cost significant sums of money—such as physical therapy. After all, these days it is not cheap and, *as the patient sees it*, it comes with no guarantee of success.

I realized that these things (uncertainty and skepticism) are the real barriers to people saying "yes." It is not time or money. And if you don't have a system to overcome this uncertainty, then they'll never pay your fees—even if they can afford to and even if they do have the time.

I realized that it was not so much about how I made their ankle feel as much as how confident I made them feel about hiring me. That is selling.

I realized that it's not so much about how good your clinical skills are as it is your ability to communicate what those skills actually do. That is selling.

It is not so much about how many years' experience you have but how many objections you can handle and then confidently answer. That is also selling.

It is not so much about how great you are at customer service as it is your ability to deal with a potential patient questioning your prices. That too is selling.

Most importantly, I realized that far from being something I should be avoiding, selling my services is something that I should be doing *for* my patients.

GET YOUR FREE SALES KIT: WWW.PAULGOUGH.COM/SALES-KIT

I believe that **selling is healthy,** and I know that if you do it right—like I'll teach you in this book—then your patients, your business, and the profession as a whole will benefit from you doing so.

I'M ALL FOR MORE CLINICAL SKILLS, BUT...

What is the lesson to be learned from my story? It is that the key to a successful and fulfilled career is not to have *more* clinical skills—it is to put the skills you do have to maximum use. That requires that you confidently sell the value of said skills so that people feel confident and want to pay to access them.

Getting clinical skills is important, but for most, the constant pursuit of another CEU does nothing but create a good topic of conversation on Twitter with other clinicians. Don't get me wrong. I'm all for getting more clinical skills as long as they're actually being used. After all, if you can't get patients to say "yes," what is the point in having skills?

Is *another* CEU in shoulder impingement really going to make all that difference when a patient questions why you don't take their insurance? Is *another* certificate in Dry Needling really going to help you when someone tells you that "now is not the right time"? Is another McKenzie course going to come in handy when a patient tells you that they can't afford you?

Sure, do your CEUs to maintain your license. But please, don't think that having more of them is going to change the challenge you're having with patients saying "no," or, just as bad, saying "yes" but only because you're the cheapest in town.

I am going to go on record as saying that the skill of selling is the greatest skill you'll ever have. It's the number one skill that you need to survive in life, let alone in business.

Having the confidence to sell what you do will attract more patients to you. After all, who wants to deal with a practitioner that doesn't even have the confidence to announce his price—let alone hold his head high when he does?

These are two of the tell-tale traits that get in the way of people saying "yes." If they get any whiff of a lack of confidence from you,

GET YOUR FREE SALES KIT: WWW.PAULGOUGH.COM/SALES-KIT

they're gone. However, if they smell someone who is confident during the sales conversation, they'll stick around. Why? Because they're attracted to the certainty that you have in yourself and they assume you're going to bring that to fixing their back problem.

STOP SELLING PHYSICAL THERAPY

As you're about to discover, to get better at selling, what you really need to do is stop selling physical therapy and instead start selling **certainty**.

Certainty is the thing that we're all craving in our lives. And when you step up and give it to your patients, they'll buy from you at whatever price you command.

There's nothing worse than spending money you think is going to be wasted. And the reverse is equally true; there's nothing better than spending money when you know you're going to get what you want. Your patients want this confidence when they buy from you.

Have the courage to see past what your peers might think and stop thinking that you're taking food off people's tables if you're asking for money. Instead, focus on sending them to bed at night certain that they're going to have their problems solved. If you do that, there's a whole new world of impact and profit waiting for you, as well as a life that is fulfilled.

I appreciate that all of this is going to go against the grain in physical therapy. But the way I see it, the way the grain is currently being sliced for private practice owners is not particularly smooth. With that in mind, what do you have to lose by at least considering that there is another way to sell your services?

The first thing you're going to have to do is get comfortable with the fact that it is okay to sell what you have to people who need it. From now on, when you sell, you're not taking money from people—*you're making them feel confident about choosing to give it to you.*

There's absolutely nothing wrong with selling someone what you can do to help them. Anyone who tells you otherwise is more concerned with how they appear to the public than making an impact on the public.

As long as you're confident that your skills can solve the problem of the person you're talking to, sell it to them with every ounce of your being, knowing that you care more about helping them than what they might think of you.

I know you will worry about what your peers might think of you for doing it, but the reality is that they're too busy thinking about their own miserable lives and everything they lack to ever think about you.

They don't like you enough to give up time that would rob time from thinking about themselves.

Don't worry about the patients, either; if someone has a problem with you for selling them *what you know they need*, it's definitely going to be a case of "it's not you, it's them." These people will have a problem with just about everyone they come into contact with—it was just unfortunate that your paths collided. You were lucky that they didn't like your approach and went elsewhere. Ideally, they went to drain the life out of your closest competitor. Why not give out their phone number just to make sure?

The reality is that most people *do* want to speak to someone who can help them make a decision. People *do* want to talk to someone who is confident in his or herself, and helps them feel assured in the decision they're about to make.

They *do* want to talk to someone who understands that their money is hard earned, but earning it is made harder by the nagging back pain that is slowing them down.

They *do* need someone who helps them decide where their hard-earned money will be spent and shows them that it absolutely will be worth it, however much they have to give up.

They *don't* want to talk to someone who looks awkward and uncomfortable the moment the money conversation comes up. They *don't* want to speak to someone who sells them a diluted version of the care plan they really need just because they're frightened of being accused of being "salesy" for doing so.

GET YOUR FREE SALES KIT: WWW.PAULGOUGH.COM/SALES-KIT

What's more, they definitely *don't* want to spend the next ten years with life-limiting back pain that they don't currently realize is coming their way.

And it's for this final reason that you being able to confidently sell your services without fear, is absolutely vital. You're going to sell what you've got so that the person you're speaking with never has to live with any of the consequences that come with *not* getting the type of great care that I'm sure you provide.

SUPREME CONFIDENCE

By the end of this book, it is my goal to get you to the point where you're living from a place of abundance and supremely confident about selling your services at the prices you should be charging.

If someone needs to buy your service, you're going to sell it to them with pride at twice the price you are right now. They're going to be happy that you sold it and even happier that they chose to buy it.

If someone needs ten sessions and they say they only want one or two, you're going to look them in the eye and tell them why your plan is a better idea and you think they should reconsider theirs.

If someone questions your price, you're going to be very comfortable with the silence that follows when you tell them that they're lucky to have called you this week, because next week the price is going up by $100.

If someone tells you they want more time to "think about it," you're going to tell them without hesitation that it is a mistake because they've already tried that—and it didn't work. You're also going to remind them that, based upon your extensive experience, time only makes back pain worse.

Running a private practice requires a certain amount of steel. It requires a *belief-in-self* that if you don't have, means you're going to get trampled on your entire career.

You've got to get used to having conversations that at first might feel awkward and uncomfortable. Though when you start, you'll soon realize that they are in fact getting you to the heart of what the patient really wants—someone who appears as certain and confident as they would expect an expert that they're about to trust with their health to be.

You can choose to get that now, or you can spend years in a perpetual state of struggle, letting everyone walk all over you, always feeling that everything and everyone around you are conspiring against you.

Believe me, this book is not just about improving your ability to sell to your patients. It's about so much more than that:

It's about you being able to sell the best staff on joining your team, selling them on your new ideas, and even selling insurance companies on the reasons they should overlook your latest admin error and pay your damn bill anyway.

But most importantly, it's about you finally rediscovering the belief in yourself that you had when you first set about opening your practice. If you've had the courage to do that, I know you've got what it takes to sell your services with ease and integrity and at twice the price you are right now.

Even if you're regulated by big insurance, I'm going to show you how to tell one or two of those profit drains to go to hell. You're going to do it just to restore some of the confidence that they've likely knocked out of you in the years you've been accepting their chicken feed reimbursement fees.

The next ten chapters of this book are going to be a wild ride. I take great pleasure in telling you that we're going to fly in the face of almost everything you've ever been told about selling and what it really takes to command the level of fee that makes being in business worthwhile.

It's with the upmost confidence and just as much respect that I say what most people in our profession believe about selling is a complete load of trash. Almost everything you've ever been told about selling is wrong and I'll prove it to you as we go on this journey to **unshakeable confidence** together.

Are you ready?

If so, buckle up and turn the page to the next chapter, where I'll share with you the most common mistakes that physical therapists make when selling their services.

BEFORE YOU TURN THE PAGE

If you have not done so already, be sure to collect the *Sales Tool Kit* that accompanies this book. Do that when you register your book at: **www.paulgough.com/sales-kit**

The Free Sales Tool Kit Includes:

- Instant download PDF containing some of the best questions you can ask in any sales situation (incoming calls, drop-offs, cancellations, etc.)

- Eleven-point checklist to make your front desk phone calls more successful

- Bonus video training of Paul teaching how to stop objections before they even happen

**Get it all, and more, here:
www.paulgough.com/sales-kit**

GET YOUR FREE SALES KIT: WWW.PAULGOUGH.COM/SALES-KIT

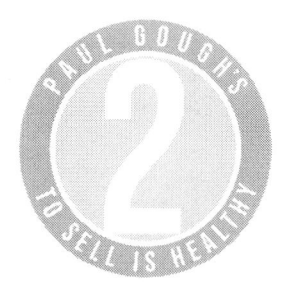

SEVEN REASONS WHY PHYSICAL THERAPISTS STRUGGLE WITH SELLING

Anytime you are speaking to a potential patient who has concerns or questions about hiring you, you're involved in the process of selling. Given that most people have concerns and questions about *everything* before they buy *anything,* it means that whether you realize it or not, you're always going to be involved in the process of selling.

How well you do it determines how many of the people making inquiries become paying patients of your practice. This is what is called your conversion ratio. If selling is the cause, then the conversion is the effect.

Most clinic owners want the conversion without having to do any of the selling. One of the reasons is because there's so much emphasis placed upon marketing it means little if any respect is shown to the need to then sell. Marketing creates what is called a "lead" (someone interested, but who has questions before they spend money with you) and the next step is to sell to that lead in such a way that they want to become a paying client.

Basically, if you want the interested person to become a paying patient, then someone has to *sell them* on why they should do so. Just because they called doesn't mean they want to book an appointment. You must separate their call from your thinking that they're going to book just because they picked up the phone.

Many clinic owners understand that they need to market their practice. But at the same time, they think that all of their problems will be fixed if they just sort out their marketing. And to a certain point, getting good at marketing *does* solve a lot of problems. But the reality is that getting good at marketing also brings other problems, such as getting

GET YOUR FREE SALES KIT: WWW.PAULGOUGH.COM/SALES-KIT

more inquiries from people who have questions that need answering before they book.

If your marketing is doing its job, then you have the *potential* for more patients on your schedule, but you still have to do something to earn it. You have to sell.

You can call it *selling the value, selling your services, selling your worth,* or *selling yourself.* They're all the same and all that matters is that someone at your practice is doing it in a way that makes leads feel confident about taking the next step with you. Someone has to be talking to the *potential* patient so that their concerns and questions are addressed. If they don't do it, you won't get the effect you want—the conversion to paying patient.

This lack of understanding of the difference between marketing and selling is just one of the many reasons why so many physical therapists struggle when it comes to selling. In no particular order, here's another seven reasons why private practice owners struggle with selling to patients. How many are happening to you?

1. TOO MUCH TIME TALKING INSTEAD OF LISTENING

If you want to influence with integrity, then you need to spend more time listening than talking. You were born with two ears and one mouth for a reason. The problem with talking too much happens because people are at their most comfortable when they're talking—and usually about themselves.

If you want to make a great first impression, the best way to do that is to stay quiet and simply listen. Think about it—why is it that you want to talk to the patient so much? It is because you're comfortable doing so. Guess what? It works the same way for them. I mean this respectfully when I say just *shut up* and let them do the talking so they can start to feel that way. If you struggle, put your hand over your mouth or cover your mouth up with tape. Either way, I recommend you shut up faster and start listening more.

I appreciate that it's a natural tendency to want to get your voice heard when someone first comes into your world. You want to get off to a good start with them and you believe the best way to do that is to lead the conversation; to talk more than them. By doing this, you think you're putting them at ease. But this can often have the reverse effect.

When you talk more than they do, it is akin to going on a first date and spending the whole evening talking about yourself. Chances are you won't get another one. The problem? When you talk too much, you're often guilty of trying to sell yourself. You don't realize you're doing it and you're not meaning to do it, but when you're talking a lot, it's a sign that you *really* want someone to understand something from your point of view. Talking too much is what you do when struggling to get them to see something from your point of view.

When it comes to effective communication, less is more. Think Twitter over writing an email. What is also little understood is that when you talk *too much,* you give people a reason not to buy. That's right, you can quite literally talk your way into objections and out of a patient saying "yes."

The often-misunderstood concept in marketing and selling is that you have to "sell yourself" to get the patient to say "yes" to you. You don't. All you have to do is listen to what they want and then explain that you understand in the context of what you can do for them. Ideally, you're doing it in as few words as possible. But it is not about selling yourself. It is simply about showing them that you know how to achieve what they want.

To do that, you've got to listen more than you talk. As a general rule of thumb, the 80/20 principle should apply. That is, they should be speaking for 80 percent of the time and the other 20 percent is you. Anything more than that and you're likely to be forcing your view of what you want onto them, or what you want for them.

Asking better questions is the fastest way to more sales success and that's why I've added an instant download PDF with my best questions to ask anytime you're talking to a potential patient for your clinic in the **Sales Tool Kit** that comes free with this book.

Get it here: www.paulgough.com/sales-kit. You will be able to use this for patients who are making initial inquiries, have concerns over price, and even when you're trying to keep them from canceling.

GET YOUR FREE SALES KIT: WWW.PAULGOUGH.COM/SALES-KIT

2. LACK OF POSITIONING OR PREEMINENCE

Positioning is about what you stand for, what truly makes you different, and how well you can communicate it. When you have it, it makes selling your services almost effortless.

Preeminence is what people believe to be true about you before they call. When you have preeminence, there's almost no selling to do because they're arriving already confident in you. With preeminence and the right positioning, patients are choosing you because they like you and what you stand for—not what you do. They've already decided to buy by the time they call you. All that you have to do is answer their logistical questions (time, cost, etc.).

By and large, private practice owners do a dreadful job of positioning and preeminence. Even when you get a referral from a doctor, what does the patient really know about you before they book? The answer is very little, and this is why even doctor-referred patients are often difficult to get on the schedule if they've got high copays or other costs to cover.

The typical positioning of a physical therapy clinic is one that is "friendly and experienced" and "prides itself on great customer service." That's fine, but there's nothing in any of that to make you different from any other option patients have. Your position in the market place is the same as the other clinics in town. You are offering the same qualities as everyone else, and that means it's hard for patients to decide. It is also why you'll feel you have to be competitively priced just to give yourself a chance of getting any patients.

Think about it. If every physical therapist in your town positions himself as a physical therapist offering "experience and friendly service," how can patients decide who to choose between? They can't. You're all the same, and so patients will struggle to choose. It means what they will actually make their decision on is the only thing that separates clinics—price. Of course, the cheapest will always win.

If you've ever struggled to raise your rates, now you know why. You might want to believe it is "your town" or that "no one wants to pay higher prices in your town," but that's not true. I had exactly the same false belief when I first started my clinic, but now I charge some of the highest fees in the country. My town did not become more economically

GET YOUR FREE SALES KIT: WWW.PAULGOUGH.COM/SALES-KIT

prosperous all of a sudden, allowing me to charge higher fees. What changed is that I positioned myself differently from everyone else and made it easier for people to discriminate in my favor.

A MARKETING PROBLEM LEADS TO A PRICING PROBLEM

A lack of preeminence is a marketing problem. To be more precise, it is a *lack* of marketing. As in, none is being done. Instead of advertising your services or qualifications, use your marketing to separate yourself from the crowd and to position yourself as an expert.

Offer health tips via a weekly newspaper column, use your social media to talk about why people in their fifties and older regularly suffer from back pain, privately publish special reports on topics such as back pain. Better still, write a book and market that you're an author on the topic.

Think about how much easier your life would be if, for example, people knew you were an author of a best-selling book on the topic of low back pain. How would that change the conversation with a patient with low back pain? You're now the person who quite literally "wrote the book" on back pain. You'd already feel more confident just because you know that they've been taking you to bed each night (by reading your book). When you're the last thing on someone's mind at night, you're pretty important to them. That is preeminence.

What if you positioned yourself in your market as "The Leading Back Pain Clinic" and everyone knew that was why you were famous? How would that change the conversation with a patient? They would show up differently and all you would have to do is find the best time to schedule them; all of the objections and concerns are answered in the buildup to getting to you, by them deciding for themselves that they want to work with you.

THE PAUL GOUGH PHYSIO ROOMS

All of the above are just *some* of the many things that I have done to create positioning and preeminence at my clinic, The Paul Gough Physio Rooms.

GET YOUR FREE SALES KIT: WWW.PAULGOUGH.COM/SALES-KIT

I wrote the book on better health. It's called *The Healthy Habit* (www.paulshealthyhabit.com or find it on Amazon). It is a book with all of the simple health habits that someone who is my perfect patient would be interested in knowing. It is marketed as "essential reading for people aged 50+" and that is because that is the age of my perfect patient. The more specific you can get, the more success you will have as more people are drawn to you.

I am preeminent and authoritative in the eyes of my perfect patient. As a result, they're more likely to arrive with fewer objections. The only time someone asks, "How much is it?" at my clinic is *after* they have confirmed that they want an appointment. They're not asking and then deciding. They've already decided they're coming; they just need to know how much to bring with them in their wallet or purse to avoid the embarrassment of not having it on them.

If your only marketing activity is a few business cards dropped into local doctors' offices, or a website that confirms how friendly and professional you are, then you'll always be in a struggle with selling to people who make inquires. That's because you're missing preeminence. You're missing a real marketing strategy.

Real marketing is about truly, (madly), deeply understanding who your perfect patient is and crafting a marketing message that promises to solve their specific problems. And then, once you know who that person is, carefully selecting the places that you share that message for it to be seen. That could be Facebook, newspapers, email, Google, and so on. Wherever you think you're going to get the attention of your perfect patient.

When you do this consistently, your marketing starts to resonate with more people. And not long after, you're inundated with the exact type of person that you love to help. Best of all, they show up with fewer objections and they're happy to pay higher fees. Why wouldn't they? After all, who else can they go to? Everyone else in town is a *generic* physical therapist trying to be a jack-of-all-trades to anyone with a pulse. I'm the authority in solving their specific problems. I'm a master of solving the problem that they've got.

What I've just described is the principle of all successful marketing and is, by and large, the entire theme of the 63,000 words I wrote in my no.1 best-selling book on marketing – *The New Patient Accelerator Method: How I Scaled A Four Location, $1,000,000 Plus Clinic (And, in One Of The Poorest Parts of The Country)*. If you have not read it yet, I recommend you do. You can get it here: www.paulsmarketingbook.com.

3. WORRY OVER WHAT OTHER PHYSICAL THERAPISTS THINK (PEER PRESSURE)

Even at the best of times, it's easy to worry about what others think of you. We all do it. But when it comes to what others think of you for selling, that really does seem to add to the worries. Add into it the fact that you're a healthcare professional and you've just intensified the worry about what others think of you by ten times.

Society seems to have labeled salespeople as being inherently bad; as if every sales-person or anyone trying to sell anything is wrong.

The reality is that it's not so much the salesperson, it's the *way* it's being done. "Bad sales" is what people hate. They hate someone being 'salesy', but they love having *someone guide them, influence with integrity and ultimately help them make a good choice*. This is the type of selling that I'm advocating at your practice.

I've heard it said that people who are in pain *should not be sold to*. I would argue that is exactly why they should be sold to. When they're in pain, they need help, guidance, reassurance, and someone to guide them more than anyone else. Anyone who is in pain today risks their entire future health on the decision they're about to make—or, as is often the case, will not make. Why should they not be sold to when selling done right can solve that problem?

With that in mind, if selling is about influencing people to make the right decision, is it not even more important to at least *try* to assist someone to make the decision to hire you? Some may disagree, but if selling ethically, professionally, and confidently is not appropriate in the situation of trying to assist someone in making a decision about their health, what is?

GET YOUR FREE SALES KIT: WWW.PAULGOUGH.COM/SALES-KIT

I agree that selling to people who do not need what you do is wrong. It is not only wrong in this profession, it is wrong in *any* profession. However, selling to people with a problem that you know how to solve is one of the best things you can ever do for anyone. I put it to you that it is wrong *not* to sell to them. What is more, we shouldn't hold back from doing it just because of what people might think.

Here's my simple piece of advice to you: if you're worried about what your peers think about you, stop thinking that they're thinking about anyone but themselves.

The likelihood is that they don't really care what you're doing, anyway. They're going to be so consumed in the lack of success in their own private practice to ever notice what you're doing. If they do happen to dislike your new sales process, it is most likely because their practice is absent of one and their doors are about to close.

They are irritated only by the fact that you are selling and marketing—knowing they never had the courage to do any of it. Their dislike of what you're doing has nothing whatsoever to do with your new website or your latest advert looking salesy. It is, however, their own unhappiness caused by a failing career or practice and they're trying to project this on you.

4. FEAR OF REJECTION

Selling exposes you to a lot of rejection simply because there's a 50/50 chance that they'll say "no" to you. When you hear "no," it's easy to take it personally and begin thinking that people don't value what you have to offer. If you hear "no" enough times, you even begin to question your self-worth. Are you as loved and liked as you thought you were? Are you as good a physical therapist as you even thought?

All of these things can happen when you're in the risky situation of having to sell. Because of that, you conclude it's safer not to do it or just accept the excuse that the patient gives you.

In any other situation with a patient, you're the one in full control. When you achieve your medical qualification, it means that for the rest of your life you can confidently stand behind it knowing that you're going to be respected for the things you say and do. This is also what many medical professionals attach their self-worth to.

It means that if you talk exclusively about things you know more about—such as back and knee pain—you're never at risk of being rejected and having your self-worth called into question. You're comfortable if you talk about physical problems the patient has.

However, put yourself in a situation where you don't feel as certain or sure about yourself—such as talking about money or cost. Having to get involved in a money or price objection makes you feel uncomfortable, and because it's not a situation in which you are expertly trained (like you are in back pain), it's easy to avoid it completely for fear of screwing it up. You know by now that screwing it up leads to that horrible feeling of being rejected.

What makes it worse is that if you hear "no" enough times, you'll soon begin to associate any and every objection with deep emotional pain and discomfort. That is not nice. Soon enough, you have a deep-rooted fear of rejection associated with the word "no" and this causes you to accept any objection that the patient gives you as fact. There's no consideration that what they are saying to you is a money problem could actually mean something else. As a result, you never even attempt to address it; you never attempt to re-sell the value of your services and so you never get good at doing it.

In case I haven't made this clear enough, the reason you accept their initial objection is not so much because you truly believe they have no money—it's the pain of you finding out it's *not* the money and that the issue is *you*. And that, at first, is worse than losing yet another patient. Said differently, it's easier to accept that money is the issue than it is to consider the idea that you might be less valuable than you think.

Please don't take any of what I've just said the wrong way. It is pretty deep. But when you stop and think about it, this is what really happens. We all have a deep-rooted need to be liked and loved and that's not something we think is possible if people reject or say "no" to us. It's why the second a patient gives us an objection we accept it as fact—even though, most of the time, it's not the real issue (as I'll show you in a later chapter).

GET YOUR FREE SALES KIT: WWW.PAULGOUGH.COM/SALES-KIT

THE FASTEST WAY TO GET OVER THE FEAR OF HEARING "NO"

The emotion that you're feeling is real, by the way. I'm not for one second saying that you don't feel pain when you hear "no." However, there is a way to get over it and here's the fastest way that I know:

Condition yourself so that whether you hear a "yes" or "no," they both make you feel the same.

It's true—the most important thing in getting over the worry of being rejected is to not get too excited when you hear a "yes," and, at the same time, not get down when you hear a "no." From now on, it is position neutral.

If they say "yes"—do not get excited. If they say "no"—do not get disheartened. Either is okay with you from now on.

You want them to say "yes," but you're not taking it personally if they say "no." It doesn't mean you get complacent and just accept their objections, but you're not going home at night feeling bad if they do. You want them to say "yes" for their sake—not yours.

This was possibly the best piece of business advice I was ever given. I would go so far as to say it was one of the best pieces of *life* advice I was ever given. I've adopted this in many areas of my life and it's helped me tremendously to enjoy the journey that I'm on growing my businesses and dealing with the highs and lows.

For example, I would like people to like me, but I'm not affected if they do or don't. I would love for you to love my books, but I'm not overly thrilled if someone says something great, much like I am not disheartened if someone says something negative. I am not labeling myself as a success or a failure in my life based upon a review of any of my books (or any of my work, for that matter). How people feel about my books or me is nothing I can control, so why would I be affected by it? I figure the only thing I can control is the way *I* feel about what I do.

If I am happy with what I've done, and I genuinely believe there was nothing more I could have done before putting my work out there, then I'm not getting affected by what someone might say. I hope that they like it for *their* sake—but not for mine.

GET YOUR FREE SALES KIT: WWW.PAULGOUGH.COM/SALES-KIT

I get the fulfillment I crave just by giving it my all. Fulfillment is a significantly better drug to get addicted to than the pain/pleasure associated with a yes or no. It's also one you can control.

This is, of course, difficult to do. Taking "stance neutral" on everything in your life needs to be worked at constantly. It's easier, though, when you understand that the reason people say the things they do are so deep and complicated that more often than not it's actually out of your control.

Whether it is the fear of losing money, looking silly in front of a husband or wife who warned you against doing it, or hearing about how their Aunt Sally got burned spending $2,000 with a physical therapist in another state or town, there are complicated reasons and false beliefs that sometimes you cannot change no matter how good you are at anything.

The phrase "you can't win them all" is very true and it applies to this situation. But I will add that it doesn't mean you can't win more than you are now. What you *can* do to start making immediate progress is to understand that as human beings we're irrational and illogical by design. You and I included. Even at the best of times, most of the time people have got no clue what drives the decisions we make.

Perhaps the best way to help you to understand this is to consider romantic relationships. Most relationships go bad and eventually break up *not* because of something that is happening in the present, but nearly always because of something in the past. What happened in the past influences how we feel in the present.

(This is deep, I know, but play along with me and keep an open mind.)

Stuff that happened years ago dictates how you react to things today; your interpretation of the world and all that is happening to you in the *now* is influenced by things that happened in the past— usually as a child.

To change how you feel in the present, you have to change how you view what happened in the past. You can never change what happened then. You can only change how you feel about it now. For example, if the reason someone is saying "no" to you today is because they have a deep distrust in healthcare people, a distrust instilled into them by their distrusting father who got deeply burned by someone in health care once—how is that anything to do with you?

If this person's father had a really bad experience, he has likely reinforced to the person you're speaking to (about three times per day for the first eighteen years of their life), to never to trust a healthcare professional like you. That is a lot of history to unravel.

Another example: if the person you are talking to has just found out that the pension that they were expecting—the one they were sold by a white-collar *professional* many years ago—is not going to pay out as much as they had hoped for, they're going to be distrusting of pretty much anyone in a white-collar role from now on.

Again, that is nothing to do with you. If they're saying "no," it is because of the distrust that someone else has caused. You're just in the wrong place at the wrong time. Why would you take that personally?

Under the banner of trying to improve your confidence, what I'm trying to say is don't take rejection personally. It really isn't you and is almost definitely them. The best things you can do are show them an appropriate level of compassion and empathy and take the time help patients to see their situations differently. Given that almost everyone has some issue or another holding them back, just imagine the impact that you'll have on them when you do.

Instead of thinking that it is about you, realize it is actually about them. It's an issue that they're carrying with them that they're bringing to your conversation. It is no reflection on you or what you charge, so don't let it affect your confidence. Ask the questions that will help them overcome their insecurities about you or your price.

5. NEVER SHOWN HOW TO SELL, OR NO SKILLS

The reality is that you're not actually that bad at selling. You've just never been shown how to do it right. You weren't that good at riding a bike until your father taught you how to do it; you weren't that good at walking until your mother encouraged you to take that first step.

A lot of people give themselves a hard time over not being very good at something, but they shouldn't. They've just never allowed themselves the opportunity to ever actually be any good at it. I think selling is the same. For all of the reasons we've discussed—such as society's dim view of selling, the professional ego getting in the way, or your physical therapy school telling you it is wrong to sell—these things contribute to you never wanting to learn how to do it.

The problem is, though, you have to do it all day, every day. There's not a single situation when you're with a patient that you're not in some way selling them. Whether it is selling them on initially buying into you at that first session, selling them on continuing to see out their plan of care, selling them to come back or giving you a referral—you're always selling.

Because selling can't be avoided, what inevitably happens is that when you're in situations that you have to do it, you mess it up. But why wouldn't you mess it up? You haven't been trained to do it right. It is simple cause and effect.

What happens next is because you feel uncomfortable and even somewhat vulnerable with selling (the sting of rejection), you never want to have to do any more of it. You start to hide from selling and spend the rest of your career convincing yourself that selling is bad or wrong or, worse, that if you just get better clinical skills then people will buy from you and the selling problem will disappear.

THE ADULT'S FEAR OF PUBLIC SPEAKING

This situation reminds me a lot of a young child who has to stand up and speak in front of her classmates for the first time. The kid dislikes the situation in the days before it even starts and when she doesn't do very well at it, she concludes that she is not very good at speaking in front of the room. The kid will spend her entire life thinking that she's not very good at public speaking and, worse, for the rest of her life tries to avoid it.

It may be true that she wasn't very good at it when she was seven. And the reason she wasn't very good at it when she was seven was simply, well, because she was seven. She'd never done it before, so how could she possibly be good at it?

If, instead of throwing her straight into a setting of having to speak in front of thirty other kids, someone had taken the time to teach her how to do it first in front of three kids, then six, then twelve, then twenty-four, within a month, speaking in front of thirty kids would come naturally and the public speaking issue that most people carry all their lives wouldn't be an issue.

The issue with selling in health care is compounded by a lot of negative views of selling, but also the fact that no one teaches us how to do it. Don't beat yourself up at this point if you're not all that good it. Well done for picking up this book to learn how to do it right.

6. NO UNDERSTANDING OF WHY PEOPLE REALLY OBJECT

Closely tied to the above, another reason why physical therapists struggle with selling is because they don't take time to understand why people *really* object.

If you think that it is only because of the price, you're mistaken or naïve at best. That is what society and the media want you to believe. They'll have you believe that no one has any money, and yet wherever I go I still see people buying things.

These days I live ten minutes from Walt Disney World and despite the prices rising every year, they can't keep people out of the parks. As for the lines at Orlando International Airport, it's a good thing I have TSA pre-check as it's never less than a forty-minute wait just to get through security.

Even in my hometown of Hartlepool in England, whenever I go back, everywhere I look I see people spending money. What I don't see is people wearing the absolute cheapest clothes, driving the absolute cheapest cars, or everyone getting the less-expensive bus option to go on vacation instead of paying more and flying.

The notion that cost is solely behind the reason that people say "no" is ludicrous; you know as well as I do that the patient who tells you "no" today is on Amazon this weekend buying the latest smart TV with the money they could have spent with you. Sure, there are some people who can't pay your fees and never would be able to, but not as many as you're currently thinking.

GET YOUR FREE SALES KIT: WWW.PAULGOUGH.COM/SALES-KIT

By and large, as a general rule, 80 percent of people are not objecting because of cost. They're objecting because of so many other reasons that they don't know how to communicate to you. There's a chapter coming up later explaining why they do this—what I call the real, underlying, root cause reasons why people object to your services. I recommend you read it like your profits depend on it. They probably do.

For now, though, I want you to start to consider and be open to the fact that what people say and do isn't always what they mean. Selling is just a way of influencing with integrity; you can never do that if you blindly accept what they say to you without prior understanding of why they're saying it.

If selling is about helping people see what you're offering from another point of view, it makes sense that you must first understand why that point of view exists. You can never be successful if you accept what you falsely believe to be a "money" thing as to why they didn't book.

It's funny how many times people have told me they can't afford me at first. Then, thirty minutes later, and with me having told them stories of how I fixed other problems that are very similar to theirs, they miraculously find the money to hire me. They didn't just win the lottery in the thirty minutes that passed while we were speaking.

No, what happened was I allowed them time to talk about their problem and then I was able to match up what they were looking for with stories about how I was able to solve that specific problem. Stories are just one way of helping patients see it from another angle. I'll teach you specifically how to do that in Chapter 5.

7. NO SALES SYSTEM

"Paul, how do I answer the, 'Do you take my insurance?' question?" This is one I get asked all the time. It is being asked as if there is some killer word or phrase that the person asking currently doesn't know of that, when they get it from me, will change the outcome every single time they're asked it.

But here's the thing: to think that sales success is all about getting a yes with some clever close or word is short-sighted. Sales success is the sum of a series of parts of a sales system that each can be optimized. In

GET YOUR FREE SALES KIT: WWW.PAULGOUGH.COM/SALES-KIT

fact, true sales success is more about what happens at the start of the call, and even how they are allowed to perceive you *before* they call, than it is what you say at the end to get them to say "yes."

Optimizing your sales system and how to do it is something I teach in my **"Effortless Selling System" Program (www.PatientConversionSystem.com/book)** and it involves you looking at every one of the touch points that the patient experiences on their journey to getting to you.

It starts with looking at your marketing. Who is the patient you're attracting, what do the headlines on your ads say, do the titles of the free information reports resonate with their challenge, what does your website communicate? Even what you say on the video that introduces yourself to them matters.

Then there's the first phone call. How is that being answered? And how can it be improved? What questions are being asked? Are they drawing insightful answers that let you engage and connect with the prospect? How much time is even being allocated to talk? Is it enough, and are they being given options of treatment sessions to pick from to effortlessly start their journey with you?

If it is a free first session, do they understand the value they're getting from that free session? Do they know they're getting $250 worth of free health care? Or did you let them believe that it was free and because of that they had no concept of the value or respect for your time, resulting in a no-show?

Assuming they arrive at your practice, how are they greeted? Are they engaged or just acknowledged? There's a big difference. Did the secretary continue the conversation about the problem they've got (that was identified on the phone) and why they're *really* in your clinic?

Or did it resort to the customary "please fill out these forms and help yourself to a glass of water from the machine" (right before closing that horrible and unnecessary glass window in the clinic waiting area)? Did they receive an official confirmation of appointment letter? Did they get a brochure with a dozen or more testimonials to read before they arrived for their first appointment? And did someone call them on the day of their appointment to get them excited?

GET YOUR FREE SALES KIT: WWW.PAULGOUGH.COM/SALES-KIT

In that phone call, was it confirmed that their real problem is noted and understood? Most importantly, was it clearly communicated to the patient that your practice *has* seen other people with this concern before?

All of these things (and more) are what goes into a sales system and every single one of them can be optimized. When you do this, it is easily the most impactful thing you will ever do that instantly boosts your conversions and ultimately your profits. If you're a solo practitioner, it's how you get away from having to do the selling. And if you've got a team of people, this is how you'll get the most from the investment you're making in those people.

Here's a key point. You might not have thought about it, but you currently *do* have a sales system. It just might not be a very good one.

However, when you get clear on this and know what is currently happening in your sales system, then it becomes easy to optimize it to improve your results. Make just ten of these touch points 10 percent better and with the compound effect working for you, you'll have a stunning improvement to your conversion ratio (that is the number of inquires who become paying patients).

If you want my help to optimize your PT clinic's Sales System, I recommend you consider my instant access program the, **"Effortless Selling System: The Complete Sales System To Double Your Front Desk And Treatment Room Conversions In Just 48 Hours"**

DETAILS:
www.PatientConversionSystem.com/book

Use The Promo Code "BOOK500"
To Drop The Price By $500.

When you order the program (which includes a physical binder that comes complete with scripts, frameworks, and training videos to follow), you will also get two free tickets to my next **2-Day Sales and Conversion Bootcamp**, where you can put all of this stuff into action with me personally!

Okay, so those are just some of the factors contributing to the lack of success when selling. Come with me to the next chapter and I'll quickly give your confidence a shot in the arm by reminding you of something very important that most physical therapists begin to overlook.

TALK TO ME AS YOU MOVE THROUGH THE BOOK:

LET ME KNOW YOUR THOUGHTS AND COMMENTS OVER ON TWITTER OR INSTAGRAM:

@THEPAULGOUGH // #ASKPG

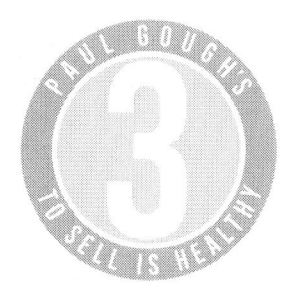

NEVER FORGET WHAT YOU'RE ACTUALLY SELLING

Never forget that what you're doing is changing people's lives. What you're doing is being done for people and not *to* them, as many people wrongly associate with sales and selling. Separate bad salespeople from the actual process of selling a vital service to people who need it. Most importantly, never feel guilty for selling.

The day you feel guilty about selling is the day you tell yourself that what you do for people is something bad. That simply isn't the case. I feel bad or apologize in situations where I've hurt people or done things that I shouldn't have; selling them on a life with better health is not one of them. I take great offense to ever being labeled as "salesy" and I am happy to let people know it if I think they're out of line for suggesting it.

I still remember a day in my clinic that I overheard one of my staff in conversation with a potential patient on the phone.

The patient in question had responded to a newspaper ad that offered them a free report on ways to ease back pain (lead generation style marketing, as explained in my New Patient Accelerator Book). The patient called, and of course the staff person who answered the phone began to ask one or two questions of the patient to uncover their real health needs and concerns.

As the story goes, my staff person was going back and forth asking him questions about his back pain. We want him to get some clarity on his situation and be in a position to give him the best advice. It's our goal with all our patients when we first speak to them.

Everything seemed fine until about twenty minutes in, when he accused the lady he was speaking to of "trying to sell to him." He said something like, "I know what you're doing here. You're asking these questions to try and to get me down to your clinic. You're trying to sell to me."

Now what happened next is really interesting. The immediate response of the person from my clinic was to defend her actions by softly responding, "I am sorry if that's how you feel, I am not trying to sell anything to you."

I AM TRYING TO CHANGE YOUR LIFE—AND YOU WANT ME TO HOLD BACK?

Needless to say, I wasn't happy. In fact, I hit the roof.

I shouted at the top of my voice that we *are* trying to sell this person something. We are selling something that will change this person's life—better health, less back pain, the ability to walk farther for longer, and ultimately a life with fewer pills and less risk of having to face dangerous surgery. For *that*, I will never apologize to anyone.

The problem here was not that we were selling to him—it's that we were doing it so well and so effortlessly that he was actually reaching the point of making a decision. When he realized that, he didn't like it.

Now why would that be? Why would someone lash out and get defensive when all we did was take the time to ask him questions and show genuine concern for his situation?

It's because of what I've already explained in the early chapters of this book: people can't and don't like making big decisions. It makes them feel uncomfortable and, in the end, they end up saying "no" to the feeling of being uncomfortable—not to the thing being offered to them. In this case, that was our services. There's even a name for it. It's called cognitive dissonance and it refers to an uncomfortable feeling you get in your brain whenever you're close to making a decision about something that is uncertain.

This person was happy to converse with my staff and answer questions right up until the point he realized that what we could do for him was actually what he needed.

GET YOUR FREE SALES KIT: WWW.PAULGOUGH.COM/SALES-KIT

It sounds strange but doing that forced him into a situation where he had to, perhaps for the first time, seriously consider spending his money and risking his time with someone to solve his back pain. More to the point, he had to consider spending time and money on an uncertain, risky service like physical therapy.

That is not comfortable. That is not a position that people like to be in. By and large, by the time they hit 40, people become what is called "risk averse." That is, they've made so many bad decisions with their time and money in the past that they do anything to avoid ever being in a situation where it could happen again. Yes, even when it comes to their health. We're not exempt from any of the basic flaws of how humans are designed just because we provide health care.

The reason many people never get the outcome or the happiness they want in life is they will never risk uncertainty in pursuit of happiness. People are naturally more comfortable accepting what they've got even if what they've got is not very much. If life is crappy, at least they know it. The worry is that it could get *really* crappy if they quit their job and pursue an alternative one.

With what they've got, they're certain with how it feels in the moment they're thinking about it and they can learn to live with it.

In the case of pain that is nagging or aching, most do learn to live with it. They limp, modify their exercise, take pills, or just pass it off as normal and part of aging. To ask them to come to physical therapy and risk losing time and money, taking clothes off in front of strange people, not to mention their view that their problem could actually be made *worse*—when you consider all of this, you begin to see why physical therapy is viewed as a risk to a lot of people.

It's a risk that most are not willing to take and that is a bigger problem for you than any economic challenge you think might exist in your town.

When you take the time to sit in your patient's shoes, you realize this is how they operate; this is how they live. It might not be how you *want* them to live but it is how they *do* live. The fact that they're in pain doesn't change it.

GET YOUR FREE SALES KIT: WWW.PAULGOUGH.COM/SALES-KIT

Remember, physical therapy is very familiar to you and I. It is not to the patient. Going to space is familiar to an astronaut. However, if you or I had to sit in the next shuttle to the moon, we would be more than a little apprehensive about it. Meanwhile, the trained astronaut next to us is pumped, excited, and loving every minute of it. It is the same situation, but we're both interpreting it very differently.

Most people's dislike of being sold to has nothing whatsoever to do with you or what you're selling; it is their own inability to make decisions on anything, made worse by the fact that they've been let down in the past perhaps by someone with a college degree just like you. And, don't forget that the frustration caused by the pain they are in can really cloud their better judgment.

When you think about it, this is why you must get better at selling. It's why I believe that selling is the best thing we can do for people. There's an argument to say that it should be the very lesson we're given at physical therapy school.

If you're bad at selling the value of what you do, patients will never make good decisions and the whole thing will always feel uncomfortable for both you and the patient.

However, when you feel good about what you're selling, they feel good about buying it. And it's when they feel good about buying from you that they'll do everything that you tell them. What is more, if they do everything you tell them, surely it is more likely that their pain and stiffness will go away? That is what you want, isn't it? That is what the profession wants, isn't it? If so, this is what needs to happen. But it has to start with you. You have to be the one who shows up with the confidence to make the person you're speaking to feel more confident about buying from you.

The purpose and need for selling is really to take away their indecision and to make them feel more secure and confident. If you do it right, it becomes an effortless situation that they don't even recognize as selling. What is more, it becomes an environment where patients *want* to buy from you. It becomes an environment in which they respect you more because you took the time to guide, influence, and help them come to the right decision to choose you.

GET YOUR FREE SALES KIT: WWW.PAULGOUGH.COM/SALES-KIT

What I'm trying to say as I wrap up this short chapter is instead of thinking that selling is something that you *do* to people, change your view to being something you do *for* people. You're trying to change their lives—don't ever hold back if you think you can accomplish that.

TALK TO ME AS YOU MOVE THROUGH THE BOOK:

LET ME KNOW YOUR THOUGHTS AND COMMENTS OVER ON TWITTER OR INSTAGRAM:

@THEPAULGOUGH // #ASKPG

GET YOUR FREE SALES KIT: WWW.PAULGOUGH.COM/SALES-KIT

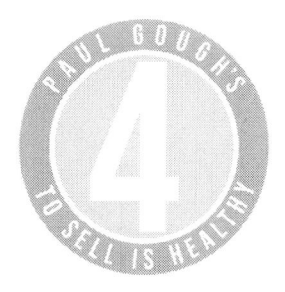

INTRODUCING "EFFORTLESS SELLING"

A few years back, I was hosting a big event in San Diego. It was my annual 2-Day Sales and Conversion Bootcamp and I'd flown in one of my staff members from the UK to be part of it. A couple of days before the event, I made my way to the airport to pick her up and when she arrived, I was happy to see her. Once our formal hellos were over, something strange happened. I didn't realize it, but I started to sell to her.

See, I'd been in the city for a couple weeks in the buildup to the event. It meant I'd already done many exciting things with my family. I'd frequented some great restaurants, spent time watching the sunset on Coronado Island, had visited places like Seaport Village and even gone whale watching a little farther up the west coast.

I was feeling good about all of the experiences I'd had—so good that I wanted my team member to feel the same way. As we headed in the car to my house, I couldn't help but talk all about each of these places and recommend she visit them while in town.

I'd had wonderful experiences and felt great for doing so. Why wouldn't I want her to feel the same way? In the moment, when describing all of these cool things, what I was unconsciously doing was selling. I was selling her on doing those things I'd already done and, crucially, had enjoyed doing.

I wasn't selling a product or a service for money in the traditional way that is often instantly thought of when the word *selling* is used. In this instance, I was selling a feeling. I'd felt great about all of the things I'd been doing, and I wanted her to feel as good as I did by doing them

GET YOUR FREE SALES KIT: WWW.PAULGOUGH.COM/SALES-KIT

too. I was selling her on doing them because I knew how great she would feel if she experienced them too.

I was selling—and yet it felt effortless. I was transferring the positive energy that I had discovered from these places from me to her.

SALES—A TRANSFER OF ENERGY

At the fundamental and most basic level, that is all that sales is: a transfer of energy. You are *trying to make someone feel as good as you do about the thing that you're selling, knowing that it is going to enhance their life.*

You've likely done this type of thing yourself—you just didn't realize you were doing it. Think about a time when a relative or a friend from out of town came to stay with you. How do you feel when they arrived? You were likely excited and happy to see them, and because they made you happy (by coming to see you), you want to return the favor by making them feel just as good.

You'll usually do that by telling them all about the things you and your family love to do in your town—the idea being that you'd like to do those things with them too. Reciprocity at its best.

They're likely to be tired from the journey. Yet, despite that, you can't help but describe the best restaurants in the area, tell stories of the places you're going to be taking them, or telling them all about things they should do while they're with you. You do it because you're sure if they do, they'll have a great time and feel equally as great for doing so.

Here's the point: if you could catch yourself in the moment when you're doing this, you would realize that all of these things make you feel good *even when you're just talking about them.* You're doing it because it makes you feel good and, most importantly, you want them to feel as good as you do. As you do it, you're selling to them.

Of course, you have absolutely no clue you're selling; you would never consider that this is what you're doing. You don't even realize that you're doing it and that you're also doing it really well. You would never believe that you're selling as you're just doing what comes naturally to you. You're not asking for money from any of them, you're simply

GET YOUR FREE SALES KIT: WWW.PAULGOUGH.COM/SALES-KIT

influencing them toward doing something you know is going to enhance their life. You're influencing with integrity.

And here is the breakthrough:

If only you would do this same thing when you speak to your patients, all of your sales problems or fears would disappear.

In case you missed it, the point I am raising is that selling is not that difficult. It's definitely not anything bad. What is more, it's actually very natural. Selling, done right, should be what I call "Effortless Selling."

Most people are doing it all day, every day with their friends and family; whether it is with a friend who comes from out of town or with a five-year-old child on why they should look forward to going to Grandma's house after school. Selling is a normal part of everyday life. It doesn't always involve taking money from people, and it doesn't always involve one person being left feeling bad about the situation. It's a really normal and natural process.

The only question we should be debating is why it doesn't happen so effortlessly in your clinic when you talk to your patients.

BEHAVING DIFFERENTLY—JUST BECAUSE YOU'RE AT WORK

The answer is really simple to explain. It happens because when most people get to work, they start acting and behaving very differently—just because they're at work.

Most people stop doing what I've just described, and this is where all of their selling problems begin. They'll take an approach to selling that is the complete opposite of what they would do to sell when they're at home or with friends.

Have you noticed this in yourself? That when you arrive at work and start to talk to a patient, all of a sudden you stop doing all of the things that you effortlessly do at home that you know will make people feel great.

The question is, "Why?"

GET YOUR FREE SALES KIT: WWW.PAULGOUGH.COM/SALES-KIT

The answer is nearly always, "Because *that is just what everyone else does.*" That is it.

I'm serious. There's this thing that has been passed on for generations that says that when you go to work, you have to all of a sudden become someone you're not; that you have to speak differently, look different, use different words, and worry more about what the client thinks of you than trying to help them.

I think they call it being "professional." You're told to be professional at work, yet no one ever tells you what that means. I'm pretty sure it doesn't mean to become someone you're not, and yet that is what most people do and ultimately become.

You change the way you act and behave at work hoping to win over the approval of your colleagues and your customers. And that's the problem—you change who you really are and so find it more difficult than it should be to sell.

I put it to you that most people struggle with selling because they focus more on *what the customer is thinking about them*, and trying to appear professional, than they do thinking what they can do for the customer.

I'm not saying you mean to do it, or are in any way bad for doing it, but I am saying that until now you probably didn't even realize that you're doing it. It feels so normal to arrive and work and think that you have to change who you are that you can't even remember the first time you did it.

Why does it feel so normal? It's because everyone else does it too. You watch them answer the phone or speak with a different mannerism or tone and you think you have to do the same.

THE CURSE: ACTING PROFESSIONAL FOR THE SAKE OF BEING PROFESSIONAL

If you can understand this concept that selling requires you to be the best version of yourself (and not some half-baked professional trying to be more professional for the sake of being professional), then you're already halfway to getting more confident at selling.

If you're not as good as you would like at selling, then I put it to you respectfully that it is because you're maybe going to work too concerned about what people think of you, or worried how you might be judged. As a result, you don't focus on or feel as good about what you sell and therefore you have less energy to transfer to the people you're talking to.

Instead of being natural and energetic, effortlessly selling people into your services with your obvious abundance and flow, perhaps you've become the consummate professional (stiff and dull), worrying about being liked and wondering if you're being judged? All of this means your energy flows in the wrong direction. It is going inward, and outward to be felt by the patient.

That is a problem because you only have a finite amount of energy; it can either go toward worrying (about what they think of you), or it can go toward making people feel great about what they're buying from you. It can't go both ways.

Instead of worrying, simply focus on being the best version of the person that you already are. Communicate in the same way you do when you're at home with friends and family, subconsciously selling things to the people that you love in the way that I described above. If you do that, I know patients will love you for it just like the people at home do.

To emphasize this point, let's play a little game:

Recall and then picture a conversation you would have with your husband or wife when you're trying to get them to do something that they initially appear reluctant to do. This is something that you really want them to do.

For example, it's Friday night and you really want to go to a different restaurant than the one your partner has chosen. How much effort and energy are in your voice when you try to persuade them to try an alternate one? How firm is your tone? How relaxed are you? How jovial? How determined are you to get the outcome for both of your sakes (because you know your choice is way better!)? What is your approach? How do you react to their initial objections? Whatever you would say, and how you would say it, pay attention to it.

GET YOUR FREE SALES KIT: WWW.PAULGOUGH.COM/SALES-KIT

Now recall and listen to a conversation you've had with a patient recently who was reluctant to hire you.

How does that sound? A little different? A little "stiff"? A little more formal? A little less casual? How is the tone? Is it fun, or is it more concerning? I bet it's the exact opposite to how you would be with someone at home who doesn't do what you initially want them to. And yet, I bet you win the Friday night restaurant argument every time.

Here's a thought: why not just do the same thing on a Monday morning with a patient who appears reluctant to hire you? However you behave at home, adopt the same strategy to win over more patients to say "yes".

After all, we're all the same. How you sell everything is how you sell anything. How you influence one person is how you influence every person. Nothing changes from person to person and it certainly doesn't change just because you're a licensed physical therapist. Be the best version of yourself and watch how many more people start to say "yes" to you.

PERMISSION TO BE YOURSELF AT WORK—GRANTED

I put it to you that to be better at selling, you don't need to change that much; you just need to change what you're doing when you arrive at work. Do the reverse of what you're likely doing right now and stop trying to be a "professional" version of yourself. Just be, well, *yourself*.

Being professional means being responsible, polite, and courteous to your colleagues and clients; it means painting yourself or your company in the best possible light. It doesn't mean become stiff, rigid, and uptight or change the way you speak in order to come across as more intelligent or important. If you're worried about what the customer thinks of you, change the customer. The right ones will love you for it.

Whatever you do, do not become someone else when you're at work. Give yourself permission to be the best possible version of yourself; to talk and communicate with your patients in a way that the people who love you, *love you to do*, and watch what difference it makes.

After all, why do they love you in the first place? It's because you are you. The reason you can do it at home is you don't really care what they think of you; you know you're not being judged by the people in your family when you do it, so you feel more *confident* about doing it.

So, let me ask you this. Is the problem with selling a confidence thing (over not being good at selling)? Or is it that you're worried about being *judged* by people and that forces you to be a different version of yourself than the one everyone else knows and loves?

Why don't you just make a decision to stop thinking that patients (and peers) are judging you and instead just get comfortable being the person you are at home when you talk to them? The person that everyone loves and likes? Either they will like you for it, or they won't. Either way, you need to be fine with it. Either way, it doesn't matter anyway. Don't link your self-worth to clients of your practice. They're important—but no one is *so* important that you should feel as though you have to change yourself.

If they do like you, great. If they don't like you, it's their loss. Cut them loose.

Through all of this, it's important to remember the that people at home (who really matter) will still love and like you. Never, ever forget that. You want patients to like you, but you only want them to like you for their sake—not yours.

You want them to like you because you have a solution to their problem and *their* life is going to be enhanced by that solution. But your life is not going to be affected if they say yes or they say no. Sure, you're going to get the fulfillment that comes with helping them, but you're not going to be made a better or more loved and liked person by this one person saying yes.

THE IMPORTANCE OF BEING AUTHENTIC

If you're still looking for a reason to do this, here's another: what people crave now more than ever is people who are authentic. They're attracted to people who have figured out how to be themselves, people who can be the same person no matter what situation they're in or who they're speaking to.

GET YOUR FREE SALES KIT: WWW.PAULGOUGH.COM/SALES-KIT

Let's face it, most people are a diluted or modified version of the person they planned to be at this stage of their life. Going to the office and having to pretend to be someone else (for the sake of someone else) is just one way this happens.

If you really do think this happens to you, and you're worried what people think of you when you're selling to them, then I want to remind you to never forget that what you're selling is going to change their lives.

(Re-read Chapter 3 if ever you forget what business you're really in—the life-changing business).

What is more, never forget that what you're selling goes way past the service you provide. It is about how you make them *feel* about doing business with you and not just what you do for them in terms of the massage or exercises you gave them. As the saying goes, "They may forget what you said. They may forget what you did—but they will never forget how you made them feel."

This is one of my favorite sayings and it's something that I've adhered to in business for many years now. It's why I am so open about saying that success in a physical therapy *business* is not so much about clinical skills; it is what you *do* for them. Of course, those things are important, but they are never as important as how you make them feel emotionally.

I believe that the feeling that they want from you is an energy or a certainty that they lack in themselves. I learned a long time ago that people go to places or buy from people who have things that they perceive that they lack within themselves.

As an example, take a look at who you follow on social media. I bet you anything the reason you do follow those people is because you believe they have something that you want—that you lack.

It is most often a level of confidence or an energy about life that you wish you could get. By following them, you feel closer to them and subconsciously believe that you'll somehow get more of the thing that they've got that is missing in you, just because you follow them. I know I do.

It's when you get to the point of changing how people feel when they're around you that you'll never have to worry about being in a sales situation. When this happens, people want to buy from you. They'll be asking what you have to sell them. If you don't like selling to people, then this is the perfect solution. Create an environment that they want to buy from.

And this is how you do it: you change what it is that you're selling. Start selling them a level of energy and certainty that is missing in their own lives. Have them buy into the energy that comes from you being aware of what it is that you really do for people—*you change their lives*.

To do that, you need to let go of ever worrying about what people think of you or how the patient might perceive you. Easier said than done. Much like I said in Chapter 2, we all want to be liked and loved. However, it is made much easier when you realize that the person who you think is judging you is actually not thinking about you at all. That would require them to actually think about someone else. People do not think about you for the simple reason that it would get in the way of them thinking about themselves.

Analyze your daily internal dialogue and add up just how much of it is spent thinking about yourself. Whether it's something you want, are fretting over, hoping you're doing a good job or worrying over being judged if you're not, it's nearly always about you. Left to its own devices, most of us spend most of our time thinking about ourselves more than anyone else. And by the way, it is completely normal. It is the way the brain has been programmed to survive.

I'm being respectful when I say it's not just you who thinks about yourself all of the time. And what I'm pointing out is your patients have exactly the same thing going on. Stop and think about it for a moment and you'll realize that no one is thinking about anyone but themselves. Here's how screwed up it is:

You think they are thinking about you; *they* think you are thinking about *them*.

You think they're judging you for being salesy; *they* think you're judging *them* for being rude when they say no.

You think they think you're too expensive; *they* think you think that *they're* poor.

GET YOUR FREE SALES KIT: WWW.PAULGOUGH.COM/SALES-KIT

And it goes on and on, all day every day. Everyone worrying about what everyone is thinking of each other, yet no one is actually thinking about anyone else at all.

There's great power in you knowing this. There's confidence to take from the fact that you know no one is thinking about you because they're programmed to think about themselves—just like you.

Here's a phrase that sums the situation up:

"At 18 you wish they would *stop* looking at you, at 40 you wish they *would* look at you, and at 60, you realize they are too busy looking at themselves to ever have looked at you in the first place."

Please, don't wait until you're 60 to let go of this feeling of being judged.

PROTECTING YOUR ENERGY

Getting you focused on worrying less and giving more energy to your patients is a vital first step in boosting your selling skills so that you can increase new patient numbers at your practice.

Sure, you still need to say the right things at the right time and present value in a way that they can understand; you still need to have your sales system optimized and follow the right scripts so that you ask and answer questions appropriately. But if you can't get this bit right, then those scripts and frameworks that I could give you would be irrelevant.

After you've finished reading this book, I will invite you to work with me in my "Effortless Selling System" for Physical Therapists online training program (www.PatientConversionSystem.com/book), but to master everything I will teach you in there, you've got to know all of this stuff first.

Before I understood the science and psychology of selling, I would describe myself as "okay" with selling and converting my patients. I wasn't brilliant, but I wasn't bad. I was just okay. But since I've added the right scripts and frameworks, I am now even better at it.

As I look back, the reason I was able to sell without having any real sales training is because I've always had an abundance of energy for what I do and what I sell. I wouldn't say it comes naturally — because it doesn't. My energy comes from knowing that what I do is going to transform people's lives and focusing on that.

I'm lucky. In my physical therapy business, I get to make people healthy and in my marketing business I get to make people rich. How good is that? When people ask me what I do, I tell them *I make a lot of people healthy and a lot of people rich.* Sometimes I do both at the same time, depending upon your definition of the two.

If you've listened to my podcast or any of my videos, met me in person, or perhaps even just from reading my books, you can likely pick up on the energy I give off. I am aware I have a lot of it. People regularly tell me it is what they find endearing about me. It is easy to think that it comes naturally or that I was born with it. But I assure you I wasn't; get me talking about politics and you'll notice that the energy is not there. I'm hardly even in the conversation if it is about something like politics.

And yet, I see a lot of people who struggle with their energy at work who will light up like a firework on July 4 the moment the conversation turns to having a debate about something like politics. When I see this happen, I often think to myself, *If only this person actually had this much energy when it came to their work. If only they would apply their energy to something they're actually in control of that can actually change their life.*

It's going on everywhere. If you look closely, you'll see people all around you wasting energy on things that don't matter, or in areas of their lives that are not going to help them.

My point? Be careful where you're spending your energy. If you're not aware of the places where your energy is lost, you'll spend your whole career losing it and you'll always struggle at selling with natural abundance.

This is likely to be the most significant chapter in the book and yet it doesn't tell you what to say or do when an objection presents itself. It doesn't give you a "killer" way of closing the sale or a "killer" way of positioning your prices to get them to buy in.

GET YOUR FREE SALES KIT: WWW.PAULGOUGH.COM/SALES-KIT

I can and will give you some of that, but it would be a complete waste of time if you do not understand and accept this basic principle: selling is simply a transfer of energy. And the real reason why so many people are so bad at it is because they don't have much energy or they're not using what they have wisely.

I PROTECT MY ENERGY LIKE MY LIFE DEPENDS UPON IT

I spend a lot of time protecting my energy. I am obsessed with protecting the environment that I am in and avoiding any situation in which I might lose any of my energy unnecessarily. I avoid conversations about stuff like politics, I do not comment on bad weather. I learned early not to spend energy on criticism. I rarely divulge my opinions on social media, I do not read the newspapers, and I certainly never watch the news on TV.

I flat-out avoid people who drain me or want to talk negatively, and I am very cautious of any conversations I have with people who, by and large, want to tell me how bad everything is.

And yes, I've even had to limit time with friends and my family for this very reason.

Just because we're family doesn't mean that I have to accept a lifetime of negativity or listening to things that depress me. What they want to talk about is nearly always stuff they can't or won't do anything about and I'm not prepared to waste valuable time doing so. Doesn't mean I don't love or care about them though. In fact, the reason I don't sit and listen is because I do love and care about them. My contribution or view of the world usually serves to irritate them and so it's best for us all to limit the time I spend with them.

If you're ever looking for an excuse to avoid one or two people in your life who drain you or your enthusiasm—whom you assume you have to spend time with—I can't give it to you. But I can tell you it is liberating when you finally stop doing it.

If successful selling comes down to how well I can transfer energy, then I must be good at protecting it. I have a finite amount of it available every day. I want it exclusively for the situations that will actually make

GET YOUR FREE SALES KIT: WWW.PAULGOUGH.COM/SALES-KIT

a difference to my life, or my family—and the people who value what I do.

I believe energy is the greatest currency on Earth. There's an abundance of money around, but there are very few people with energy. When you are around someone with it, you want some of it from them. It is contagious. You want to be in their presence more and more and this is what you have to be striving for as you live your life. Best of all, it's a decision you can make right now. Will you?

TALK TO ME AS YOU MOVE THROUGH THE BOOK:

LET ME KNOW YOUR THOUGHTS AND COMMENTS OVER ON TWITTER OR INSTAGRAM:

@THEPAULGOUGH // #ASKPG

GET YOUR FREE SALES KIT: WWW.PAULGOUGH.COM/SALES-KIT

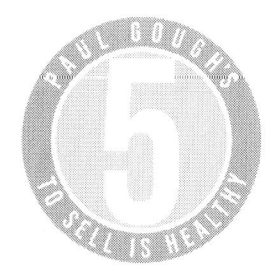

THE THREE MOST IMPORTANT ASPECTS OF A SUCCESSFUL SALES PROCESS

Once you've got your energy taken care of, and you're aware of how that makes people more likely to want to buy from you, the next thing to consider are the three things that make up the Sales Success Triangle.

These are the three fundamental rules of selling *anything* and are as follows:

1. You have to get clear on **what** you're selling

2. You have to get clear on **how** you're selling it

3. You have to get clear on **who** you're selling it to

Here's how they all fit and work together:

FIG.1

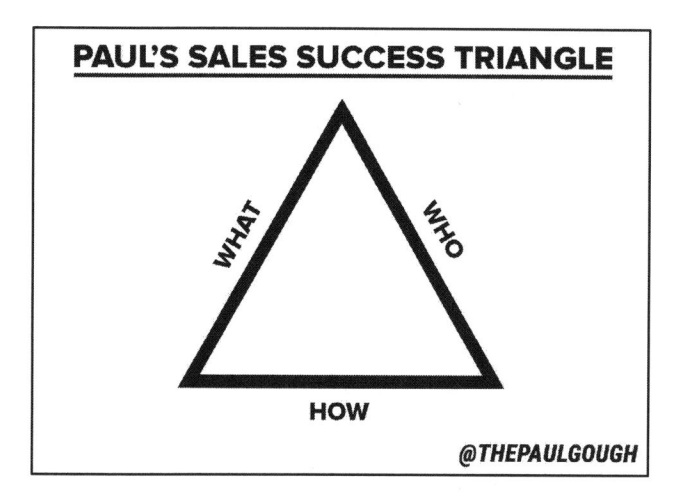

PAUL'S SALES SUCCESS TRIANGLE

(Triangle with WHAT on left side, WHO on right side, HOW on bottom)

@THEPAULGOUGH

GET YOUR FREE SALES KIT: WWW.PAULGOUGH.COM/SALES-KIT

1. WHAT YOU'RE SELLING

You may provide physical therapy to people. What you trained to become is a licensed physical therapist; the sign on your clinic's door might even say physical therapy. But what you really *do* for people is something much bigger and much more important to them than physical therapy.

What is that? Well, the short answer is, *it depends*. That is because ultimately what you do for the patient will always depend upon what the patient wants you to do for them.

Every patient wants something different and the most important skill is being able to apply your clinical skills to achieving the outcome they desire. It starts with working out what that is and not just assuming it is pain relief or restoring function.

I believe the *best* thing we can do for them is what they want us to do. In that respect, what we do as physical therapists is open to much debate. It is not defined (or limited) by easing pain or increasing their ROM. Nor is it limited by giving them exercises or pre-rehab. Reality is a construct and so is the value of physical therapy.

It starts by separating what *they* want to achieve from physical therapy and the actual process of doing the work required by a physical therapist. They are two very easily and often confused things. Meaning, separate the massage and exercises from their ability to walk or get back to playing golf. We *do* the former, but they *want* the latter.

Most people in our profession label themselves as physical therapists and in doing so *limit* their definition of what they do for people to being just that—physical therapy. It's as if the skills and the process of doing massage, prescribing exercises, or diagnosing problems are the defining factors. But that's not strictly true. Your career will not be defined by how many skills you have—only how you use those skills to help people get what they want.

In that respect, the only thing you can sell is the outcome that they want. The only obstacle to you selling more is how well you can find out what they want—what they really, *really* want—and then communicate that you know how to achieve it with the skills you've got.

GET YOUR FREE SALES KIT: WWW.PAULGOUGH.COM/SALES-KIT

But it is never about selling the skills or even physical therapy, it is never about selling your credentials, and it is never, ever about your experience, like many assume. For proof, when was the last time you asked a pilot of the aircraft you were getting on how many years he'd been flying the route you're taking? When was the last time you popped your head inside the cockpit and asked, "Have you done this before, Captain?"

I know you think that they do, but people's *actions* tell you that they don't value experience all that much. What they do is take for granted that you've got it and that is because most of their time is spent on thinking about getting the outcome; i.e., what they're going to do when the flight lands in Orlando and they get to Disney World.

So the million-dollar question is surely this: "How do you find out what your patients want you to sell them?"

Well, the answer is really simple—you ask them. But the thing is, you can't just ask, "What do you want?" If you ask that, they'll tell you they want their pain taken from their knee. Sure, that is what they want. But it's what is behind that, such as the fear of risking knee surgery or losing independence, that we've got to discover. You'll do that by asking what I call value-based questions that get to the heart of what they really want from you.

It's why you must get the resource PDF that accompanies this book. It gives you some of my top questions to ask during any sales conversation you're ever going to have with a patient and is available here: www.paulgough.com/sales-kit. Until you ask people, you'll never know what they really want, and you'll always be thinking that what you're doing for them is physical therapy.

I know it is what you want to sell them, but anyone can do physical therapy for them. Anyone can talk about their muscles, ask them for a pain score, or put a piece of plastic against their knee and measure their range of motion.

It's *only* when you've found out that they want to be able to get back to hiking again (because it's their weekly source of good conversation with dear friends) that you should stick that plastic goniometer against their knee and take the ROM reading. The number on its own is largely irrelevant; it might get you reimbursed by the insurance

GET YOUR FREE SALES KIT: WWW.PAULGOUGH.COM/SALES-KIT

company as you justify treatment, but it doesn't do much to get someone to buy into your services in the first place.

Just for fun, here's a "typical" conversation that you might hear in the treatment room between a physical therapist and patient:

Physical therapist says: "Oh look, this plastic thing shows your knee only bends to 93 degrees of flexion *and* you're missing 6 degrees of extension! This means you need physical therapy. Let's start with 11 sessions."

Patient says: "All that sounds interesting... but I only came in here to see if you could help me walk along the beach with my dog without my knee hurting. I'll have a think and let you know about that offer of physical therapy. In the meantime, I'll look on YouTube for some exercises."

It's a typical conversation but it isn't a good one if you want to help more people. Do not overlook the simplicity of what I am saying here.

And I know you're thinking, *But I do take the time to listen and I do ask them questions.* I am sure you do, but I am wanting you to be aware of how likely it is that you are talking more about things that are familiar to you than them. It's a natural tendency to want to speak in the language that you're familiar with. Adjusting that is a skill that needs to be honed.

SELLING IS NOT TELLING

Highlight this next line: *selling is more about asking than telling.*

I used to think that I had to *tell* the patient what they should do or what I was going to do. As if I was the one medically trained and they should do as I say. But that's not how it works. You've got to lead them to where you know they need to be by asking the right questions.

It's easy to think that you're giving away your authority when you ask them what they want, but you're not. You're displaying empathy and the confidence to hand over the decision-making power to the patient. You know that what you're asking is leading this person to where you know they need to be. This is a skill you must master.

GET YOUR FREE SALES KIT: WWW.PAULGOUGH.COM/SALES-KIT

All of the questions you ask must make the patient feel as though they're in control. That is what matters most. It's not who is in control—it is who *feels* in control. And it must always be the patient. In the case of life or death heart surgery, the surgeon must be in control. And the patient must feel like the surgeon is in control. But this is not life or death. They're choosing a service that they know very little about and one that is going to cost them a lot of money. It's for those reasons they must feel as though they're in the driver's seat throughout this process with you.

It is for that reason that I say that I don't do physical therapy; *I do whatever the patient tells me that they want to achieve.* I will ultimately sell whatever the patient wants to buy.

If they want to be able to walk farther with less back pain, I'll sell them that.

If they want to be able to play golf twice a week and enjoy a beer at the 19th with their buddies, I sell them that.

If they want to be able to get in the CrossFit box so that they can get back to doing their WOD, I sell them that.

If they want to be able to play soccer with their grandkids without waking up the next day with a swollen knee joint, I sell them that.

If they want to be able to get down on the floor with their kids—and actually get back up again—I sell them that.

I'll simply use my physical therapy skills to achieve the thing that I am selling to them.

The key point here is that I'll use the same skills as you perhaps would, I'm just more likely to get a faster buy-in and for twice the price than you charge for doing this, and all I am doing is what they want me to.

2. HOW YOU SELL IT

How you sell it refers to the direction you take when presenting the reasons for what you do—and why they should buy. For example, will

GET YOUR FREE SALES KIT: WWW.PAULGOUGH.COM/SALES-KIT

you *tell* them they should buy, or will you *show* them why they should buy and let them decide for themselves? Will you insist, or will you guide them toward the point where they want to buy, asking the right questions along the way?

Will you try to use logic ("the research says") to help someone make an emotional decision (not losing independence)?

Will you talk more about your credentials and experience, or ask more questions about them and their concerns? Will you quote the "evidence" from the latest course you've taken, or will you tell more stories about other people who you've helped, who are just like them?

To do it with ease, it needs to be the latter.

Asking great questions and compassionately telling stories is the secret cocktail mix to how you sell successfully and without worrying about coming across as salesy.

Here's why it works:

People love to talk. They feel comfortable doing it and they are even more comfortable talking about themselves. What is even better than talking about themselves? It is talking about themselves *when they're in pain.*

Think about it, who do you know that doesn't love to tell you all about their latest ailment or pain?

It is the easiest thing for anyone to do. And the easiest way to facilitate that situation between you and the patient is to ask questions—and then simply shut up and listen. Even better, take notes on what they're saying so that they can see that you're actually interested.

Why does taking notes (with a pen and paper) work? Simple. Think about how many people are not listening to them right now.

Their husband or wife doesn't understand how bad it is. Their colleagues are sick of hearing about their latest aliment, and the kids would only be interested if it was posted on social media. Basically, no one is listening to them about this thing that is really important to them.

Why don't you be the first one to do it?

Give them every possible ounce of your attention and allow them to talk for as long as possible about it; you want them to tell you everything.

BECOME THE OPRAH WINFREY OF THE PHYSICAL THERAPY PROFESSION

You should aim to be like Oprah Winfrey interviewing a troubled guest for her TV show; eagerly anticipating every little thing that they're saying, emphasizing your facial expressions every time they mention somewhere that hurts, and empathizing deeply as you confirm that you heard the words, "And no matter what I do, it just won't go away."

Okay, I'm joking. You don't need to become Oprah. But you get my point, right? Let them see that they've been heard.

Here's the best bit: whenever they stop talking, assume that they've got something else to tell you. When it goes silent, stay silent for an extra second and watch what happens. I guarantee that they'll start up again. It is the universal law of life—people are not comfortable with silence, so what they do is start talking again whenever they're in silence.

By the way, as an aside, now you know why so many people talk so much trash; they don't like silence so they just keep talking even when they have nothing good to say. Try it with your friends. When they stop talking, just stay quiet and then watch how much rubbish they talk after the period of silence is over.

This is a really groundbreaking strategy I am teaching you here. It's called "just shut up and listen." Even when you get to the point of thinking they've said all that there is to say, it's still worth saying, "Tell me more." Then, after they've finished, say, "And anything else?"

Let them talk themselves into feeling comfortable with you so that they start to trust you more. I know they'll do that faster if they hear the sound of their own voice. They're comfortable with their own voice—yours is strange. They've been told all their lives by their mothers not to trust strangers, so don't expect them to override that just because it is you. Let them talk for long enough and their brains begin to feel comfortable in the environment that they're in with you—and more likely to say "yes" to you. It is not rocket science, is it?

Imagine if one of those expensive physical therapy schools taught you this in the first year of starting your expensive degree. Don't you think we'd all be able to help more people? I know I often bash the physical therapy schools and I hope it *does* come across that I am; I'm baffled by their ignorance when it comes to not teaching us how to actually understand the people we have the skills to help so that we can help them more.

When you do this, you'll get to the point I described earlier in the chapter where you'll find out precisely what your patients want and what their struggles are. Then, and only then, will you be able to match up what you can do to help them with what they want from you. Do this and you'll be in a league of one. You won't have any competition—even if there's a clinic right across the street from you.

Your competition is selling physical therapy from a clipboard and asking questions from an EMR. Meanwhile, you've become the Oprah Winfrey of the medical world, *empathizing* with your patients like only Oprah can, taking the time to custom-tailor the perfect solution for them when no one else has taken the time to even ask if that's what they want.

TELL ME MORE

Just to make sure you've got this, here's how your next new patient evaluation or front desk phone call needs to go:

"I'm sorry to hear that, *tell me more…*"

"And what else…?"

"Really, that *is* interesting, anything else?"

"Sorry to hear that as well. Tell me more about that."

"I'm so pleased you told me that. What else do I need to know?"

Just keep asking!

GET YOUR FREE SALES KIT: WWW.PAULGOUGH.COM/SALES-KIT

If you remember nothing else from this book, remember this phrase: "Tell me more." Aside from "I love you," they're the greatest three little words that you can ever say to anyone. Do this today and when you do, pay attention to your patient's reaction. Watch their face light up when they realize that you *do* actually care and you're not treating them like a billable unit, like most healthcare places do.

THE IMPORTANCE OF STORY TELLING IN SELLING

The other thing I mentioned earlier, under the banner of *how* you sell physical therapy, is something that all of the best companies on earth do well—they story tell around their product.

Telling a story is the most natural thing on earth to do, and yet most physical therapists never consider doing it when they're talking to their patients. People enjoy stories; they feel safe in a story. My little boys love it when I tell them a story. I do so every single night before bed and any other opportunity that I get to do so. In fact, I love to tell stories just as much as you likely enjoy reading them, so why don't I tell you a story about how my two boys love me telling them stories. Ready for the story?

So whenever we are by a swimming pool—on vacation or just at our house in Orlando—one of the things that my eldest boy, Harry, loves to do after he's finished in the pool is sit next to me on my sun lounger and hide us both underneath his towel so that no one else can see us or hear us.

He then says to me, "Will you tell me a story, Daddy?" And of course, I oblige. When I do it, I realize it is in *that moment* I have something special; I have his absolute and undivided attention. When I am telling him a story, over and above any other situation, he is listening to every single word I am saying.

Now one of the reasons for that undivided attention is the story I tell him is always about him and his day. It always starts with "Once upon a time, there was a little boy named Harry."

In the story, I will always recall how *his* day started and what *he* has done in his day so far and I do that so that he can find himself in the

GET YOUR FREE SALES KIT: WWW.PAULGOUGH.COM/SALES-KIT

story. I want him to know *he* is the main character in this very special story. After that, I just make the whole thing up as I go along.

I may bring into the story *his* favorite Disney characters or the superheroes *he* sees on TV and the story wanders off to wherever it goes. What matters most is not what the story is about, but the fact that *he* is in the story. If at any point I forget to mention that *he* is involved or *he* hasn't heard *his* name for a few minutes, then he reminds me to do so.

As the best stories do, at the end, the story always finishes with "and they all lived happily ever after." He literally finishes those words with me every single time.

Here's the point of the story: at five years old, no matter what the storyline, Harry wants the story to be about him. He wants it to be relevant to the things that are important to him in his life right now — things like Mutant Ninja Turtles and Power Rangers—and he wants it to finish with a happily ever after.

Well, guess what? So do your patients. *They* want a story that features *them* and that ends well. Why don't you tell it to them?

They will feel safe in that story and because you're not at any point talking about you or selling your services, they're listening without any negative bias or preconception.

Best, much like I do with Harry and Tobias, my other son, you have their full attention. They're listening and hearing. It's rare that you get both and there is a difference. When you tell people stories, there's no resisting what you're saying, and they are able to understand much better if you say it through a story.

Storytelling also bypasses the guard that the brain puts up whenever it's in an uncomfortable situation. When you go to buy something—anything—your brain knows that doing so comes with some element of risk; that you could lose time or money. Instead of absorbing all of the information needed to make a good decision, because it is lazy, the brain prefers to block out information so that you feel less likely to buy.

It doesn't mean you don't need it or want it. It just means that your brain is lazy and it is trying to protect you in the easiest way it knows—by keeping you from making a decision.

However, if you sell through stories, you bypass this. You get past the gatekeeper, if you like. Think about the gatekeeper who protects you from getting to the doctor you want to speak to about getting some referrals. In the physical therapy profession, that person is usually referred to as "that dragon in reception."

Her job is to protect the doctor's time. She's usually good at it to and does so by blocking people who might waste it (i.e., physical therapists coming in wanting to tell him how good they are and why they should get all of his referrals). You don't like that she does it, but she's just protecting the doctor from harm. The brain basically does the same thing.

How do you get past that "dragon" at the front desk? Well, you're unlikely to do it with your killer clinic newsletters. But you might do it with your cookies and cakes; the newsletters are logical, the cookies are emotional.

It is from the emotional part of the brain that people do things like buy physical therapy or let you in to see doctors. Stories also get patients emotional. Stories also get people to do things that they otherwise appear to not want to do, such as incur out-of-pocket costs for physical therapy.

AN EXAMPLE OF HOW YOU MIGHT SELL THROUGH STORY

This is so important that I want to spend a bit more time on this and give you an example of how you might sell through storytelling.

Let's say a guy named Bill, who is 55 years old, calls you up. He's got chronic low back pain, he has suffered on and off for over a year, and he tells you he wants an appointment. He's interested, but like most people, first he has a couple of questions about what you do and how much it costs.

At this point, you now have a choice.

Option 1 is to directly answer the questions he asks. You can tell him how qualified you are, that you're a licensed physical therapist, and that you are able to fix his back pain and that your costs are $250 per session.

GET YOUR FREE SALES KIT: WWW.PAULGOUGH.COM/SALES-KIT

Option 2 goes like this: you acknowledge that you've heard his questions and subsequently explain that if you first ask one or two questions of your own, then you'll be able to give better answers to his questions. Ultimately, you'll give him the best information to make the best decision (that isn't just based on money or insurance).

If you do the latter, it allows you to take the time to ask why he is calling, what activities the back pain is stopping, and, crucially, discover something really important: why he's waited so long to call you.

Assuming that you do all that, you quickly discover things about this person to allow you to start building your story. He tells you that he's a keen golfer, he's got back pain that is causing him some discomfort when he swings, and it gets worse when he gets halfway around the golf course. He's at the point where he has had to stop golf completely because the next day's pain and stiffness is too much to take.

Right now, everything that matters to him is on hold. Not just his golf or his handicap improving, but his social circles, the friendships, his fun, his exercise, his camaraderie, and the ability to get out of the house for two afternoons per week to have beer on the 19th hole with his buddies. Because, after all, it is the latter that golfers enjoy the most!

Now, because you now know all of this about Bill, it allows you *tell a story* that is perfect for him—just like the one I tell Harry when he gets on the sun lounger with me after being in the swimming pool.

How do you start your story to the patient? It is really simple, and it goes like this:

"Bill, let me tell you a story...."

Seriously, it doesn't get any easier than this. Simply take the time to ask them a few questions about what they are really calling you for so that you can match it up with a *story* for them to find themselves in. One that, of course, has a happily ever after.

It might go something like this:

"Let me tell you a story, Bill. There's a guy who I've just finished helping. He is a keen golfer, he is also in his fifties. He used to play with a handicap of 10 and it was getting progressively worse because of a long-standing back issue that he'd been trying to cope with using pain relief pills.

"He came to me about six weeks ago telling me that whenever he hit the golf ball hard, his back pain would strike so sharply that it would cause him to misplace the ball every time he hit it.

"In the end, he struggled to get the ball to land on the fairway. It was getting so bad that after eight or nine holes, he couldn't walk without having to constantly sit down and lean over to stretch his back out. He got the point where he would have to stop and face the embarrassing situation of having to get a golf cart to pick him up from the course and take him back to the clubhouse.

"He waited three months before calling me because he assumed that his back pain would get better with rest. It never did. I remember he told me that his pain went away when he wasn't playing golf—but as soon as he went back to hitting the ball, it returned. That's why he thought he would just keep giving it more time.

"Anyway, thankfully he found me and eventually came to see me. We worked together for a few sessions and I was able to get him back to playing golf within just a couple of weeks—pain free.

"In fact, he sent me a text message earlier today saying he had hit his first hole-in-one in years and that he's loving being back on the 19th—where the beer is served.

"I know most golfers who call me tell me it is the golf they miss—but I know *secretly* that what they're missing is the social aspect of it and I'm so glad that I've been able to help so many male golfers in their fifties restore not just their handicap, and ability to play golf again, *but the ability to get out of the house a couple of times per week and away from the wife and kids to be able to goof off with their buddies!*

"Isn't that what you really play golf for, Bill?"

There you go. *That* is the story that Bill needed to hear. It was a story that he was able to find himself in and featured all of the things that he is currently thinking about, worrying about, or secretly wanting and it finished with a happily ever after.

GET YOUR FREE SALES KIT: WWW.PAULGOUGH.COM/SALES-KIT

Believe me when I say this: when you are able to do this type of thing with all of your patients, you won't have many sales issues. I've been doing this for more than ten years and it is the most important tool in my belt when it comes to getting patients to confidently buy into my services.

When people are confused about what to buy or who from, one of the things they do is go to places where other people with similar problems have been. It doesn't have to be their friend or anyone they know, they just need to know that someone with concerns similar to theirs has been to you before.

In this case, when I started talking about the 19th hole, golf carts, hitting the ball straight, hitting a hole in one, and any other phrase that is the language of a golfer, that person comes to their own conclusion that this is where people like him come. They hear familiar language and their brain feels safe as they've heard those things before in places that they trust and feel good.

It works because your brain shortcuts making decisions if it hears familiar language; it drops its natural tendency to want to protect you as it recalls other situations that you've been in where you've heard this language before. Because of that, it can conclude that it is safe. The patient starts to feel safe, and if they feel safe, they feel comfortable. And if they're comfortable, they're going to buy.

When you talk to them like this, in a language that is familiar to them, any questions they have after you've told the story are just validating the decision they've already made. Sure, they might still ask the price (logical), but it is just to make sure they've got the cash or money on the card when they arrive.

Selling isn't that difficult; it is, however, complicated by people wrongly trying to sell themselves. As I've said many times, that is not what you need to do. You need to find out what they want and then sell that.

How you do it is through asking the right questions and then telling a story of a past patient just like them, with health struggles, hopes, dreams, and fears, just like them.

GET YOUR FREE SALES KIT: WWW.PAULGOUGH.COM/SALES-KIT

When you do that, they'll listen without prejudice and they'll come to their own conclusion that you're the one—the only one—who understands them and knows how to solve their problems. When they reach that conclusion, they're in; they've bought into you and what you can do for them. And the need to sell (as people wrongly understand it) is gone.

One tip for you is to start writing down stories that match up to the five to ten most common types of problems you get in your clinic. And by problems, I don't just mean back or knee pain. The real problem is what that pain stops; it could be golf, CrossFit, Pilates, being at the swing park with kids, being unable to care for their husband or wife—whatever it is, have a story in mind for the next time someone calls you.

All you have to do is recall what the last person really wanted from you and tell it from the point of view of how you understand what they're going through right now. If you do that, they'll assume that you've done this before and they're one step closer to buying from you.

3. WHO YOU'RE ACTUALLY SELLING TO

The third and final aspect of successful selling is the *who* you're actually selling to. You cannot and should not try to sell to everyone. The situation that you're shooting for is that you are only ever selling to people who *know, like, and trust you*.

That is achieved by effective marketing that identifies a pocket of people whom you believe you can help, then using different marketing media to show them how you can help them. It is not to advertise your services, it is to market highly specific solutions to highly specific problems that this pocket of people are living with on a daily basis.

You can rarely get far in a conversation about sales without talking about marketing. If you're constantly picking up the phone to talk to people who start the conversation with "Can you tell me how much?", it is a good sign that you're not attracting people who know anything about you. Your marketing is not being seen. That is going to make selling way more difficult that it needs to be.

Most clinics' sales problems are compounded by the fact that they don't do any marketing; what they do, if at all, is actually advertising.

GET YOUR FREE SALES KIT: WWW.PAULGOUGH.COM/SALES-KIT

Let me explain the difference.

Advertising is where you tell people that you're a physical therapist, that you have a clinic, and tell them how to get in touch with you. The problem? It's all about you. It's all about what you do and is not about what problems you solve for people.

Rule number one of successful relationship marketing (which I advocate) is that it's about them, their problems, and showing them that you know what problems they live with. When you do this, they come to their own conclusion that you're the person to solve their problems for them. They're now buying and there's little selling to do.

As I said in Chapter 2, most physical therapists have no positioning or preeminence and this is why they hear the "How much?" question so quickly and frequently. For people to *know, like and trust you,* they must have had some prior experience with you before they call.

Ideally, they've been on your email list having requested a free report, they've read your columns in the local newspaper, they've watched your video on Facebook, or they've interacted with you at a local community event. This is how you'll increase the *know, like, and trust* aspect of the person calling you.

ARE THEY EVEN HELPABLE?

The other thing to consider is this: is the "who" you're currently trying to help even the right "who" you *should be* trying to help?

It's a very serious question. Is the type of person you are currently marketing to the type of person you can help? Not everyone wants to be helped or can even be helped.

Most healthcare professionals naturally want to help anyone and everyone. But here's what is fundamentally wrong with that: not everyone is actually helpable. And for anyone to be helped, they first must *want* to be helped.

Have you even considered if the "who" you're marketing to is willing and able to pay the fees that they will need to in order to get the help you want to provide? I know most people rarely consider either.

Being able means have they got the funds to do so and *willing* means that they actually want to spend it with you.

What might surprise you is that the most important is not whether they are capable—it is whether they are willing.

Access to cash is important, but not nearly as important as being willing to spend it. After all, when did a lack of cash ever stop anyone from going on vacation or buying new clothes that they couldn't afford?

This is perhaps the most important question that you'll ever ask yourself in your business. I spent five years in professional soccer working as a physical therapist. Despite the vast knowledge and expertise I had in the sports injury field, there's a reason I didn't come out and start a sports injury clinic as everyone assumed I would.

That reason was the fact that not many amateur sports players (weekend warrior type!) are willing to pay to restore their health. They're just nowhere near as committed to fixing an ankle or hamstring sprain as I need them to be and certainly not in the way that the "who" I picked really is.

It's why at my clinic, we specialize in helping people aged fifty plus live with less pain, maintain independence, and live free from painkillers. That is not to say we don't treat people in their thirties—of course we do. We just spend more time and focus on marketing to someone in their fifties and above. Almost all of the Paul Gough Physio Rooms' front-end marketing is designed exclusively to talk to someone in their fifties and above; doing that lets us talk specifically about the problems they've got so that we can get them to buy into us before they've even called us.

Here's why it works. First of all, it means we'll actually get our marketing material watched and read. If you're aged fifty or older and I put out a video called "Critical Health Mistakes Made by People Aged 50+ And How to Avoid Them," it is likely that you'll watch it.

Secondly, it makes us more appealing than any other option they've got. If we're talking exclusively about the problems experienced by people over the age of fifty, and my competitors are talking about themselves (credentials and experience, etc.), we will get the call over them every time.

GET YOUR FREE SALES KIT: WWW.PAULGOUGH.COM/SALES-KIT

Even better, it means we don't have to do much selling because they've likely done one of the things I mentioned above, such as read one of my newspaper columns, read my book *The Healthy Habit* (positioned as "Essential Reading For People Aged 50+"), have watched a Facebook video, or received emails from me talking all about the issues they're living with.

That means they've already bought into what we do and how we can help them. Which is, of course, solve the specific problems that they're living with.

Anyone in their thirties or below may still come to see us, but we're not going to try all that hard to sell to them. If they're asking the "price question" continuously and it's obvious that they know nothing about us, I wouldn't want them to book that appointment yet. I'd much rather that they take some information from us and *then* call back next week and ask any questions they might have.

But trying to get someone over the line who doesn't know anything about me—that is not what we do. I don't want their business at any cost. I want their business on my terms and at my prices, otherwise it is more hassle than it is worth. After all, the phone is continuously ringing with inquiries from people aged fifty and older who do know about me and who have already bought into me.

It is the same in my marketing business; clients often tell me the names of other clinic owners who they think that *I* should be calling to sell them my programs. No matter who tells me to do it, I never do. I simply tell the client to tell their clinic owner friend to start listening to my podcast, buy a book, or watch my videos on YouTube with the instruction that if they like what I have to say, they should call me.

If they like me enough, they'll find my number online. If they don't like what I have to say, they won't call me. Either way, we both win. In every situation, I accept that I can't and don't want to win them all.

MY BUSINESS MODEL

My business model has for a long time been about staying small with big profit margins. Some people want many clinics and that often comes with smaller margins, but they're going to sell for a big amount later. I respect that. But for me, what I want from my clinic is cash flow.

I've built it to be a free-flowing cash asset that produces money for me every month. I have no plans to sell out. I want the profits *now* to spend on good times with my kids or re-invest into starting other businesses (such as the real estate business I have recently established that buys two-to-three-bedroom family homes and rents them back out to produce yet more cash flow).

Cash flow is the real king.

That is a strategic decision I've made and what matters is not what you want—*it is that you know what you want*. My business is compact and smaller than it could have been, but it's very profitable and I'm very happy with it.

How I achieved it is more important that what I achieved, if you're looking to copy me in any way. I did it getting very clear on *who* I am selling to and figured out how to be the *only* solution to solve *their* specific problems. Despite all of the other physical therapists in town, I'm the only one they're going to choose. Doing so also means they will pay me more than they would any other physical therapist.

So, there you have it—three big aspects of selling that you cannot overlook. Next, let's look at one of my favorite topics, the *predictably irrational behavior* of your patients when they're in a sales situation with you. Turn the page and prepare to be enlightened.

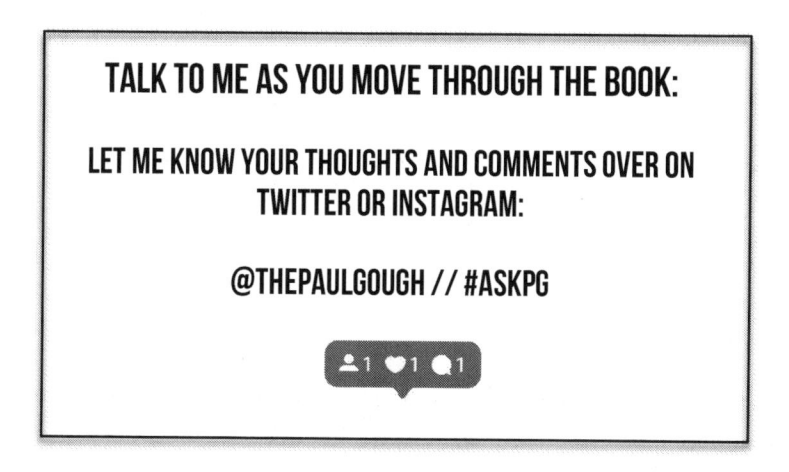

TALK TO ME AS YOU MOVE THROUGH THE BOOK:

LET ME KNOW YOUR THOUGHTS AND COMMENTS OVER ON TWITTER OR INSTAGRAM:

@THEPAULGOUGH // #ASKPG

GET YOUR FREE SALES KIT: WWW.PAULGOUGH.COM/SALES-KIT

GET YOUR FREE SALES KIT: WWW.PAULGOUGH.COM/SALES-KIT

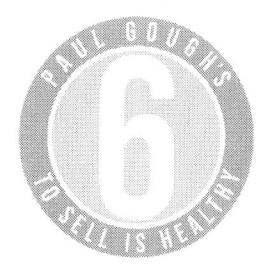

WHY PATIENTS REALLY SAY "NO"

Broadly speaking, there's only ever one reason that people say "no" to hiring you and that is a lack of trust. This lack of trust causes patients to *feel* like the investment they need to make with you is a risky one and so they'll tell you it's something like money or time.

It's nearly always thoughts that create feelings, and once a feeling of doubt is created (because of a lack of trust), what they'll do next is tell you something like you're too expensive or money is the issue. They do that to protect themselves from an impending bad decision.

But it is rarely about the actual availability of money; it is almost always how comfortable they are spending it. If you don't believe me, just look at how much debt people are in right now. They feel so comfortable spending it that they're willing to borrow it to get whatever it is they want.

My point? Money isn't the underlying issue. They can get their hands on it if they want to. Most actually have it to spend, they just choose to spend it elsewhere. If they're not willing to spend money with you like they are other people, it's because they don't feel comfortable doing so. There's distrust that is getting in the way.

And that's what we're going to cover in this chapter. We're going to look at the four causes of distrust that lead people to feel like they have to tell you it's a time or money thing instead of saying "yes" to you.

1. LACK OF TRUST IN THEMSELVES

Most clinic owners assume that the reason the patient is saying "no "is because of them or their prices; they take "no" personally and rejection is taken to heart. They never stop to consider that sometimes, many times in fact, the root cause of the distrust actually has nothing to do with them and is more to do with the patients' distrust in *themselves.*

Think about the typical life of your typical patient; by the time they've reached a certain age (usually 40), they've been burned by so many bad decisions they doubt that they can ever make a good one again.

Having made bad purchase decisions in the past—whether on a house, a car, a partner, a marriage, or some kind of monetary investment, even trivial things like clothes or holidays—they're-battle scarred from doing so and are inherently scared to make any others.

· The lack of trust is not your doing; you haven't necessarily caused it, but at the same time you haven't done anything to help them overcome it.

The other obvious scenario that is very real and needs considering is that many of the people you're speaking to are not the primary decision-maker in the family. As such, they don't know how to make decisions even if they have the cash in hand. They may not have been burned in the past simply because they've never been in a position to make any decisions in the past. They've never felt what it is like to get burned and suffer the consequence of having made a wrong decision.

You will likely know someone who has lost their husband or wife and the person left behind really struggles to cope without them. They're not only grieving for their loss; they're literally lost in the world without the other person because the other person did just about everything for them; including making all the major decisions, or they made them together.

Making decisions is a muscle that you flex. If you stop using a muscle in your arm for thirty years, it is going to waste away. It is no different with decision-making. Stop doing it and expect the ability to do it to fade away.

2. A LACK OF TRUST IN YOU

So, if it's not them, it has to be you, right? Well, bluntly, yes! Distrust in you is very likely. Not to be taken personally, but very plausible. After all, you're a stranger. And the patient's mother has most likely done what your mother did to you and conditioned you to not talk to strangers. After hearing it every week for the first eighteen years of their lives, why on earth would they trust you?

Having a patient start by distrusting you is 100 percent normal. It is the way that people start out with everyone new they come into contact with. But that doesn't mean that they have to stay distrusting. Often, the only difference between them distrusting you and then later trusting you is time.

Time is so simple and yet it is so often overlooked in business—and is especially overlooked as a solution to sales and conversion problems.

Think about how fast we expect people to make big decisions on spending money with us. Sometimes patients make the call to your clinic at 9 a.m., and by 2 p.m. that same day they are being asked to spend hundreds or sometimes thousands of dollars with you. Very few people are comfortable with doing that for anything.

Know this: if something is under $100, it is classed as an impulse decision and there's less pain and less risk associated with the purchase. That means it can be made right there and then without hesitation. However, anything over $100 is classed as a "non-impulse decision," meaning that there's often more time required before the purchase is made.

THE FORTUNE IS IN THE FOLLOW-UP

That is why I say that the "fortune is in the follow-up." I happily accept that people often need time before they'll buy, and I build my clinic and optimize my sales system accordingly.

In reality, knowing this forced me to change my business model and my pricing. It meant I had no choice but to price my services at an appropriate level so that we could afford to give patients all the time that they need to make decisions.

To get them to buy in, we need to spend twenty, thirty, forty (and more) minutes with new patients when they call the clinic or walk inside. There's really no other way to get them to buy into the clinic before they get to the clinic—at the prices I want to charge.

Most clinics could never dream of spending that much time with a patient because they don't have the staff to do it. They don't have the staff because they can't afford to pay them. But they can't afford to pay them because they don't charge the prices to make the profit needed to pay them. It's a vicious cycle.

Because I'm priced appropriately, it means I can staff appropriately to meet my patients' fundamental basic buying needs—not just their physical needs when they get into the treatment room.

It's not about whether they can afford you. It's always about the time you can afford *them*. I've had situations where people have walked into my clinic and started the conversation having zero intention of hiring us on that day.

I know because they start the conversation by saying something like "I'm not ready to book an appointment I just want some information." They lead with the "I'm not ready to book" to protect themselves. By saying it, they feel they've bought some immunity from us selling to them or putting them under pressure.

However, we've learned that just because they say they don't want to book it doesn't mean they won't. We know it's all about asking them the right questions and if they're still there some twenty-five minutes later, we've discovered that they do want to book an appointment. If I didn't have the appropriate level of staff, we'd lose this patient. By keeping this patient, I can afford to pay the staff. It's a positive and self-fueling cycle.

This never surprises me anymore. It's simply a trust thing. At first there's none of it. Twenty-five minutes later there's enough. Just keeping asking questions to keep them on the phone or in the clinic. Charge enough money to provide the level of service that people actually want to pay for.

A LACK OF TRUST ALSO REDUCES MARKETING RESPONSE

This lack of trust also explains why your marketing may not always hit it out of the park the first time you try.

GET YOUR FREE SALES KIT: WWW.PAULGOUGH.COM/SALES-KIT

Here's what usually happens when owners start to market. The typical clinic owner only markets because they have to. Usually they don't like doing it, they don't want to do it, and it's a begrudged use of their time. It means they do the absolute minimum to market and it usually involves one-off ads that the owner runs to "see if it works."

Of course, with that attitude, it rarely does. There's no multi-step approach or twelve-week campaign mapped out in advance that considers the fact that you're basically a stranger when you first enter a new media or someone's newsfeed on Facebook.

If they're seeing your ad for the first time, particularly when you're promising things like improving health, it is natural for them to be skeptical at first. Why wouldn't they be? They've suffered for years. They're trying every possibility that they can get their hands on with poor results and all of a sudden you appear promising a life happily ever after without pain. Their initial reaction is obviously going to be one of disbelief.

But, with time, and having seen you in the newspaper for a couple of consecutive weeks, they begin to trust you more and feel more confident with calling you. The ad didn't change, their back pain might not have changed. What did change was their level of trust because time got in the way between the first time they saw you and the day they decided to call you.

Each time they saw you, they felt a little more comfortable and your face became a little more familiar. This builds the trust that is missing in the beginning. So, is the marketing issue really a marketing issue, or is it that you want it to work faster than maybe your patients are willing to move because they don't trust you?

Candidly, this happens to me all the time. When I first put out my videos for people to watch on Facebook, I know full well that people don't initially like me. I know that their initial reaction was "Who is this spammer", (perhaps you did it to me too?), or some variation of it. I also know, though, that had nothing whatsoever to do with me or my videos. It is simply that my videos and I are new and unfamiliar to the person whose newsfeed I am in.

However, because I understand this, it doesn't deter me from continuing to market. I know that if I keep putting my videos out,

GET YOUR FREE SALES KIT: WWW.PAULGOUGH.COM/SALES-KIT

eventually people will become familiar with the videos and will decide to click and watch one. And when they do, it doesn't even end there. When they first click to watch the video, they might not like my voice. Why would they? It's new.

But then the next day, when the same video arrives again in their newsfeed, they press play again and all of a sudden my voice seems a little more familiar. Why? Because they heard it yesterday. And so it goes on and on. The only difference between my videos being liked or not being liked is often time.

It is the same for you when you first put out your content on social media. You're being received in the exact same way.

I honestly believe that the reason my marketing is way more successful than most others is because I understand and live by this principle. When most clinic owners are scared and anxious about a lack of ROI after the first day of an ad going out, I am trusting in the process and letting nature take its course while adding more steps to the campaign to maximize its success.

Time cures a lot of things and this is certainly true in the case of marketing a physical therapy clinic—and choosing a physical therapist.

HOW PEOPLE INTERPRET WHAT YOU'RE SAYING

Another thing that causes a lack of trust has nothing to do with what you say to people but *how* you say it and how you *appear* when you're saying it to them.

When you're communicating with a patient, only 7 percent of the message they're getting from you comes from "what" you actually say (i.e., the words and the order in which you use them). The rest of what they pick up from the conversation, and ultimately make their decision on, is based on your body language (how you hold yourself) and your tone of voice (how you say what you say). It is weighted significantly in favor of your body language; the thing that they can see. It means you can't just obsess over what to say. It's actually more about how you look when you're saying it and the tone you're using when you're saying it.

GET YOUR FREE SALES KIT: WWW.PAULGOUGH.COM/SALES-KIT

As I look back on my career, I would say understanding this was the first moment where I felt things really changed for me. I can still remember the day it happened. I was travelling from London to Bali to meet a friend of mine who was travelling solo around the world. I was working as a soccer physical therapist at the time and was moonlighting in the evenings seeing a few private patients after the players had gone home.

It was the end of the soccer season and I had seven weeks off, so I decided to head out to Asia to meet my friend Ben. At that point, I wasn't what I would call an avid reader of personal development or business books. For some reason, though, on this particular day I decided to pick up a book from a store at the airport just before my flight. I knew I had a nearly twenty-four-hour journey ahead of me and I knew my iPod wouldn't last the full flight.

I picked up this book on persuasion and influence (I name the book and author in the Sales Tool Kit you get free when you register this book: **www.paulgough.com/sales-kit**) and from the minute I started reading, I never once put it down. I was hooked. I couldn't believe that I hadn't heard or been told about things of this nature before. I read the whole thing on the flight and couldn't wait to get back to my clinic to implement everything I'd learned about how to talk to people, how to sit authoritatively, how close to get to people, and even how to look them in the eye and for how long.

These are all significant things I was never aware of that were contributing to how patients would perceive me and if they would hire me.

It was at this same time I discovered other things about how people really buy. One fact that stood out to me was that at the time of making a purchase, what people buy is a *perception* of what you do for them—not what you actually do for them.

When you hand over money to anyone for anything, in that moment, you rarely get the thing you bought. Instead, you're getting a perception of what you want. Think about buying clothes: you have them in a bag, but you don't get the feeling of the new clothes being on you (the thing you actually bought) until you wear them.

GET YOUR FREE SALES KIT: WWW.PAULGOUGH.COM/SALES-KIT

If you're purchasing a flight that doesn't take off for weeks after you paid for your ticket, what you actually bought was the *perception* that it will get you to where you want to be at the time you need to be there.

If it is a hotel, you bought the perception of a good night's sleep. But you don't have the end result yet, despite handing over the money. You only bought the *perception,* and it happens whenever you purchase something.

HOW DO YOU APPEAR TO PATIENTS?

With that in mind, I want you to think about this: how do you hold yourself when you're talking to a patient? Do you sit upright confidently and look the patient in the eye as you talk? Or do you slouch awkwardly, looking constantly up and down at the floor, unable to maintain eye contact for any period of time?

Whatever you do, you should know that your patients are picking up on all of this information. What's more, they're using it to decide how confident they think you are and then making a judgment on how much they trust you based off how much you appear to trust yourself.

If you don't hold yourself with the posture of someone with confidence, they'll begin to have doubts about you and that shows up as distrust. You'll hear it as "no" or "it's a money thing."

You've likely done this yourself too. We've all had experiences with a doctor or a dentist who, when you look at them, doesn't look like you wish they would—someone *confident* when diagnosing what ails you. Yet, what they're saying could be the best advice for your concern.

But if *how* they say it is not supporting your view of what an expert looks like—and the level of confidence a so-called expert should have—it will appear in the form of distrust. Because they didn't *look* confident, you will have doubts in the back of your mind about whether the advice you've been given was even correct. You have nothing to support that thought other than how the person looked and spoke. If it is true in those situations for you as a patient, it is just as important in your conversations with your patients.

GET YOUR FREE SALES KIT: WWW.PAULGOUGH.COM/SALES-KIT

To get more people to say "yes" to you, you've got to be considering how you look at people, how you walk, how you sit, how you shake their hands, how you maintain eye contact, and even the tone of your voice. Like it or loath it, these things *are* being factored in when a patient makes their judgment on whether they trust you or not. It is not just your credentials or experience or how many certificates are on the wall in your clinic.

Fun exercise: if you've got physical therapists who work for you, take a closer look at their body language, examine how they hold themselves, and listen to how they talk to patients. I bet you anything that the ones who have the highest number of patients on their schedule are the ones who walk and talk like *they know* they know what they're talking about. Whether they actually do doesn't matter as much as they *think* they do—and that the patients feel the same way.

3. LACK OF TRUST CAUSED BY YOU BEING TOO CHEAP

Gasp! I bet you weren't expecting to see this one in here! The idea that you're too cheap and that causes distrust is very real. This is one of the excuses patients will *never* verbalize to you but it does cause a level of distrust when someone is making a purchase decision.

Think about it, who wants to hire the cheapest healthcare professional they can find? In fact, when was the last time you went to the cheapest dentist, doctor, or nurse you could find? Who do you know that is searching Google right now looking for the cheapest physical therapist to take their kid to or have their sciatica checked? Sure, there might be one or two, but they're certainly the exception and not the norm.

I put it to you that for many people reading this book, one of the reasons they're losing patients is because they're just so cheap and so underpriced that their value is instantly questioned.

I have no doubt you've done the same thing as a consumer.

You go shopping for a new TV and you are adamant you're going to buy a certain make and model. Just as you pick up the box with the TV you want, you notice one that looked like the one you're picking up, but it is priced at $500 more. When this happens, you instantly begin to

GET YOUR FREE SALES KIT: WWW.PAULGOUGH.COM/SALES-KIT

question *what is missing* from the cheaper one that you originally wanted.

Seeing the more expensive ones throws you into a spin while you try to work out what is so wrong with the one you were thinking of buying. You want to know why the other one is more valuable. Of course, there might not be anything wrong or even different about the cheaper one, but the price causes you to think that way.

The price changes how you *feel* about your purchase. It causes you to second-guess and doubt it and you're naturally drawn toward wanting to know what the more expensive one has that yours perhaps doesn't. You subconsciously become less trusting of the cheaper one and more trusting of the expensive one—just because it is more expensive.

Price is a statement of value. It is *still* the easiest way to differentiate between things, and yet it is rarely considered in private practice when setting prices.

If you're telling me you're one of the best physical therapists in town, with amazing skills and credentials, and yet you're charging bargain-basement prices, then there's an obvious disconnect between what you believe and your reality. That is something that will be *felt* by patients.

When you claim to be the best and charge so little, do you know what you really are? You are too good to be true. And if something is too good to be true, people have doubts about it as they've all bought something for really cheap that they thought would be great—and it turned out it wasn't.

I don't know anyone who is the best at what they do and yet charge the least amount of money. If your prices are "middle" or "average" even "fair," congratulations—you've just labeled yourself as "average." That is great, but don't then try to kid anyone that you're the best.

Cheap is about *acceptable* quality, average is about *okay* quality, and paying higher prices gets you closer to *top* quality. What do you provide?

If what you do is top quality, charge top-quality prices. If you're offering Ritz-Carlton service, charge Ritz-Carlton prices. Don't kid yourself or your patients that you're offering them Ritz-Carlton service but will only charge them Motel 6 prices. They're not daft. It's not possible to do it, and they'll think you're too good to be true. They'll think something is wrong.

I don't know where your prices are right now, but I bet they're lower than they could be. Every clinic owner I work with starts that way.

Every year at my 2-Day Sales and Conversion Bootcamp, to get clinic owners to realize just how low their prices are, I play a fun game with the attendees. I ask all of the clinic owners in the room to stand up and then sit down when I shout out the price point they charge. I start at $100, then go up by $50 increments.

You would be amazed at the faces on the people who are sitting down when they see clinic owners from their town still standing up and charging one hundred to two hundred dollars more than they are.

Seeing and knowing that others are charging more than you is a powerful driver to raising your rates. It's why I would encourage you to come to the next 2-Day Sales and Conversion Bootcamp. I'll work with you personally on raising your rates and I'll show you others who are already doing it. You get two free tickets to the two-day event when you enroll in the **Effortless Selling System Program** that is available from here: **www.PatientConversionSystem.com/book.**

I'll end this point by reminding you that people choosing you just because you're cheap is not a great way to run a business. How does it make you feel to know that you're getting the nod just because you're the cheapest physical therapist in town?

That last sentence might irritate you—and I hope it does. It might give you the candid "kick-up-the-ass" you need to raise your rates to the level that is appropriate for the impact you have on people's lives.

LIVE WITH A LITTLE SWAGGER

Let's get these prices of yours to a level that screams self-assurance and supreme confidence in what you do and what you're about. Your patients will pay you for feeling that way. That is how they want to feel, too.

When it comes to health, it is *that* person people want to hire. It's the one with supreme confidence and assurance that is felt from the get-go.

They do not want the one with most credentials or CEUs. They have no clue what any of them mean. They want the one who makes them *feel* the most certain and secure in their decision. After that, then your credentials and CEUs come into play, but your level of certainty and confidence—your swagger—must come first.

After reading this book, I want you to have a little more swagger. And don't worry what other people think when you swagger around your clinic or when you're dominating social media. Remember, they're not thinking about you anyway as they're too busy consumed by themselves wondering what's missing from their own lives.

The good news is that you don't need to wait to fill up your schedule or wait until you're a "bit more experienced" to give yourself a pay rise. It is a free market. Even if you're regulated by insurance, raise your rates on all of the things you charge cash for and start dropping one or two of the worst-paying insurances. Do it just to make to make yourself feel good.

Send them a "go to hell" letter (see Chapter 10 on what to write) knowing you're replacing $50 reimbursements with $300 per session patients who will pay you up front. It's great for cash flow and the soul—not to mention your swagger.

Finally, you might be thinking that if your prices are low that will mean more people will say yes to you. And it might be true. But that would also be the worst thing that could ever happen to you. That is because charging low prices means you're also going to be very tired, struggling to make a profit, and, yes, you might even have a wait-list—but that is only because you're the cheapest they can find on Google. Again, how does it feel to be cheap?

4. LACK OF TRUST IN THE OUTCOME

The other obvious thing that affects trust is the patient not being sure that they will actually get the outcome they want. You might be certain they will achieve a full recovery from their simple low back pain, but it's a different thing altogether for them to feel the same way.

As I always say, it is never about how we see it, it is only about how *they* see it; it is never about what we want for them, it is only ever about what they want for themselves. Meaning? You have to see it from how they see it for them to ever consider moving forward with you.

What we do comes with an uncertain outcome. No matter how good you think you are or how good you say you are, there's always a chance that the outcome will not go as expected. You can't fix them all. It's just the way it is in health care. People need certainty in their outcomes much like they need to know when things start and when they end. Whether they're watching a movie, getting on a flight, or driving to the beach for the weekend, your patients know when everything starts and when it's going to end. That is not always the case with physical therapy.

One of the massive mistakes I've seen physical therapists make on the phone or in a consultation is to tell patients something like, "Let's start with a few sessions and see how it goes." That's like getting on a flight and the pilot saying, "I'll take off and see how it goes when we get up there." If that happened, you wouldn't be very confident about the pilot and you'd likely want to get off before takeoff.

HAVE THEY BEEN LET DOWN BEFORE BY ANOTHER PHYSICAL THERAPIST?

The other thing that makes them distrust in the outcome is the obvious one—they could have been let down by another provider somewhere else. If that has happened, it is tainting their view of you.

Just as bad, they might not have had physical therapy themselves, but they know someone who has but who didn't get the outcome they expected. If they know someone who has a dislike of physical therapy, that person will have created a seed of doubt that causes distrust in the outcome. You've now inherited that problem.

The key is to recognize it. You can't change their bad experience with physical therapy, but you can acknowledge it and help them see it differently. One of the first things I do is to re-frame it so that their past bad experience becomes a good thing that is going to help us to solve the problem faster.

GET YOUR FREE SALES KIT: WWW.PAULGOUGH.COM/SALES-KIT

I might say something like, "I know you didn't get the outcome you expected last time, but now we know what doesn't work for you, that means it's going to be easier and faster for me to find what does work for you."

This is a great line I would use whenever I spoke with a patient who has distrust in the outcome from being let down by another provider. Never criticize or bad-mouth the other providers as you're just creating more distrust in the decision—and in physical therapy.

Make them feel good for what they did in the past; congratulate them for going to see the last therapist and remind them how much that is going to help you as you work together to get the solution.

> **TALK TO ME AS YOU MOVE THROUGH THE BOOK:**
>
> **LET ME KNOW YOUR THOUGHTS AND COMMENTS OVER ON TWITTER OR INSTAGRAM:**
>
> **@THEPAULGOUGH // #ASKPG**

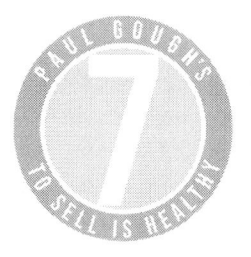

PRICE IS NOT THE PROBLEM

Telling someone what you charge is difficult. The words come out of your mouth and you hope and pray that they are fine with them. You tell them what you charge, and you sit and wait in a proverbial state of worry over whether or not they'll find the fee acceptable. You hope that you haven't offended them, and you wonder if they're judging you for being greedy for asking for such a high amount. At the same time, you hope that your price is just low enough to be accepted and yet not too high as to be rejected. Sound familiar? If it does, it's how most clinic owners feel and think when they're talking about price.

You would be forgiven for thinking that your patients think and feel the same way as you about the amount you charge—but the reality is they don't.

It's very likely that the only person concerned with the price is you.

You would also be forgiven for thinking that $100 means the same to every person that you talk to—but it doesn't. It can't. That is because we each have different thermometers when it comes to money and that is why you must let go of what *you think* the amount you charge means to the person you're talking to. It can't possibly mean the same to everyone.

For example: your fees might be $200 per session and seeing that might make one person feel uncomfortable and yet the next person feels completely fine with it. Thus, the actual amount is not the problem. It is only how they *feel* about it.

Another way to look at it is like this: let's say the total cost of hiring you is $1,000. That might make someone feel very uncomfortable at the thought of paying it, and yet previously they have spent $1,000 on a new TV and felt very comfortable doing so. From this, we can conclude that spending $1,000 is not the problem.

GET YOUR FREE SALES KIT: WWW.PAULGOUGH.COM/SALES-KIT

It exposes the only other issue. That is *what* they are spending that $1,000 on and how they *feel* about it. When it comes to the price, it is always how they *feel* about what they are spending their money on. And ultimately, that is determined by how they're *allowed to feel* by the person asking them to pay that price. In this case, that is you.

Let me explain in more detail.

In the last chapter, I explained how *distrust* is the root cause of the reason people say no to hiring you. Well, depending upon the level of distrust, it could cause a *mental* discomfort known as cognitive dissonance. It's a real feeling and it's likely already happened to you multiple times this week.

It is this cognitive dissonance that surfaces when people hear that your fees are slightly higher than they were expecting to pay for physical therapy services. It doesn't mean that they don't want to pay or can't pay—it just means they're feeling a little uneasy about the prospect of doing so. They're uncomfortable about spending more money than they have in the past on this type of thing. The bit that is so important is when I say, "on this type of thing." And what I mean by that is their issue is not spending $1,000. No, their issue is spending it on physical therapy.

But the actual amount isn't the issue.

You will have felt this cognitive dissonance yourself on many occasions. It is an unpleasant sensation in your brain that makes you *feel* physically uncomfortable when you're thinking about buying something. It usually happens when deciding on things that come with some level of perceived risk or loss (i.e., physical therapy).

When you experience it, if the level of intensity gets to a certain point that you don't like, it causes you to do and say things to escape the feeling; things such as "I can't afford this" or "Now isn't a good time."

The feeling acts as a warning signal to cause you to think more carefully about the purchase before you make it.

For example, you're thinking of buying a new laptop. You start to look online and your initial budget is $1000. As you search, you find one that is out of your budget by $500. You start to think about whether or not you should buy it (even though it's over your budget) and as you get closer to doing so, the more that this sensation called cognitive dissonance kicks in.

The more you think about buying it, the stronger that uncomfortable feeling in your brain gets. In the end, it is this uncomfortable feeling that causes you to close the internet browser and decide to come back to look at a later date.

This unpleasant *feeling* is what people move away from—not the price. Not the actual amount.

Now what this feeling also does is stops people from getting to the point of considering what the value of the thing is. That's a problem, because this is what we need to consider if we're ever going to buy something that is priced higher than we expected. It stops your patient from thinking long and hard about whether they really can or can't afford it, if they really will get value from it, if they want to give up something else to be able to get it, and even asking questions that will give them answers to ease how they feel.

And this is where it becomes relevant to you as a physical therapist.

Any time we have to make a decision that comes with some level of risk, this sensation of cognitive dissonance comes on. It gets worse the bigger the risk and it mainly happens when there are conflicting attitudes, beliefs, or behaviors about a particular thing. In the case of buying a new laptop, it could be, *I know I can't afford this...but I've worked really hard lately, so I deserve it.*

In the case of a patient deciding on physical therapy, they could be thinking, *I know I need this—but what if it doesn't work? This is a lot of money to lose if it doesn't work.*

This is a conflicting belief. One that produces a feeling of discomfort and crucially leads to an alteration in your patient's belief about what money is available to them. This is why people who you just know have the money say they *don't* have the money.

They're not short of money or being tight with it, they're actually under the intense pressure and genuine pain caused by cognitive dissonance. It is this pain in their brain that is causing them to change their own beliefs about what money is available to them and ultimately leads to them telling you they can't afford you. They are changing their behavior in order to reduce the discomfort they're feeling.

Basically, when cognitive dissonance kicks in, it is easy for patients to forget that they paid more to fill up their Bentley in your parking lot than you're asking to fix their low back pain.

The thing to remember is what I said at the start of this chapter—that your $1,000 fee is not the issue. They're comfortable spending that amount on a cruise or on a TV. The issue is that physical therapy has an *uncertain outcome*.

It is the uncertain outcome component that is causing the dissonance leading them to feel uncomfortable about your price. And that is what causes them to change their belief about what time or money is available to them. *This then changes their behavior and they will decline coming for any more treatment.*

This doesn't just happen in physical therapy. People change their beliefs and behavior about things all the time thanks to cognitive dissonance. Let me give you a few examples from scenarios I am sure you will have experienced from some of the people in your own life:

1. **People who smoke** know it's really bad for them and could actually kill them. They know that to be true and that makes them feel uncomfortable about smoking whenever it is pointed out. But what a smoker might do to quickly make himself feel better about the fact that he *could* be slowly killing himself is say something like, "Well, you've got to die of something—might as well be something I enjoy." They're able to change their belief about smoking and so too their behavior (i.e., they keep smoking)—and, crucially, how they feel about it. In this case, they lose the dissonance and continue to do it.

2. **Someone who has just bought a new, more expensive car than they could afford.** This person *knows* they can't afford the extra $20,000 it costs and that makes them feel uncomfortable living with that extra debt. But they wanted the car. That uncomfortable feeling after they have bought it is the fight between wanting it and not being able to afford it. This is dissonance at work. To move away from it, this person will alter their attitude about *why* they bought it in the first place. They'll

have to come up with some reason or say something to stop this pain. And it's usually something along the lines of "safety."

The next time your friend or neighbor tells you that they bought their new car "for the kids because it has a great safety record," you know that they've likely bought a more expensive car than they can afford. They are altering their belief that the car is a required purchase because it is "safer for the kids."

They can live with their purchase if it is for that reason—even if they can't pay the mortgage.

3. **When your sister or best friend calls and tells you that she's booked a two-week vacation to Hawaii**, you know she can't really afford it when she says "We've worked so hard this year" or "We really deserve it after everything that has happened in the last few months." Basically, they feel uncomfortable about the debt they're now in (that was required to pay for the holiday) and they need to alter their belief about why they bought it or did it in the first place.

PEOPLE DO BUY THINGS THEY CAN'T AFFORD

What's all this got to do with physical therapy? It's this—right now, I suspect that you currently think people make rational, responsible decisions about their time and money from their own free will. You currently think people only buy things that they can afford; you currently think that they can't have their decisions swayed; you currently think that people cannot have their belief about what money is available to them altered.

I've just proven to you in three very different examples that they absolutely can change their belief and behavior—all you have to do is help them do it so that *both of you benefit*.

It absolutely *is* possible for someone to buy something that they say they can't afford. It *is* possible for people to alter their beliefs about what they're buying and the value of it. And *you* are in control of this—not them.

The critical thing to understand here is that in all of the circumstances I described above, they're changing their beliefs and attitudes about money in favor of a certain outcome.

Cigarettes give an instant hit of calmness; the new, expensive car gives an instant feeling of getting one over on the Joneses living next door, and the expensive vacation to Hawaii brings an instant hit of excitement knowing that they're going to a new destination.

The problem with physical therapy? As we've discussed, there's no instant hit and no certainty in the outcome. All roads lead back to a *lack of certainty in the outcome.*

Left to its own devices, cognitive dissonance works against us physical therapists. In these three examples, the person is altering their beliefs in favor of buying or doing the thing because the hit—the outcome—is 100 percent certain.

So how can knowing this help you become more confident when selling your services at twice the price you are now? Well, once you know what the real problem is that is causing them to say no, it is much easier to overcome.

The obvious and perhaps only solution to this problem is to afford your patients more time. If you want them to figure out how to afford your prices, you've got to figure out how to afford them more time.

Time is the gateway to helping them feel more comfortable about your prices. The typical clinic barely keeps the patient on the phone for any longer than three minutes. You can't possibly expect them to process the value of the price you're asking for in this short amount of time.

It is why I will forever bang the drum for keeping patients on the phone or in your clinic for as long as you can. If it's the first phone call, I insist on my staff spending at least twenty minutes with new patients to ensure they're as comfortable as possible before they arrive.

You do that by asking what I call value-based questions that increase the depth and length of their answers. It is also why I suggest you never answer the "How much do you charge?" question without first asking one of your own. The more time that you can spend with someone making them feel comfortable before you get to talking about money, the more trust you will build *with* them and the less cognitive dissonance will build *in* them. Do that and you'll get them to the point that they want to change their belief about what money they have available and this time it'll be in your favor.

RECOGNIZE WHEN THEY'RE FEELING UNCOMFORTABLE

The real, blunt truth is that people are not necessarily short of money or time, they just feel uncomfortable in the moment they're talking to you about giving you either. Because of this, they don't know what else to do or say to ease it other than to tell you that money is the issue. And this is the lesson I am hoping you'll take from this chapter, that people do not have an issue with your price as much as how the price makes them feel. And if you let that feeling take control of the conversation, you'll keep losing the patient.

The key is to recognize when a patient is feeling uncomfortable and do everything you can to take them past this phase; to take them to a place they're thinking more rationally, able to see that what you're asking for is actually less than an amount they've spent in the past. Replace their doubts and fears with certainty and assurance, and buying physical therapy becomes as easy as clicking to buy a HDTV from Amazon Prime.

If you want to win their business, you have to win their trust. It's *your* job to mitigate how they feel about the risk that comes with hiring you.

What is more, the more that you charge, the more you'll need to control this. Do whatever it takes to help them see your value proposition differently. Ultimately, sell them on what you can do for them in a way that makes them feel as certain as buying a car or going on vacation.

From now on, instead of being uptight about their reaction to your price or accepting their automatic answer about the cost being too high, I hope you'll be able to confidently *change* the conversation and start to say things like, "I *understand* you're feeling a little uncomfortable right now," or, "I can sense that you're *feeling a little uneasy* about this situation. Is it because you think physical therapy might not work for you?" After all, this is precisely how they *do* feel.

Do this, and you've just become a real expert in their eyes, an expert in solving the real problem that they've got—indecision (like I first spoke about in Chapter One).

In almost every case with a patient who tells you money is the issue, the real issue is that they simply feel uneasy about the price of an uncertain outcome and they will do or say anything to get away from that feeling. The emotional pain of indecision is nearly always worse than the physical pain in their leg that they've called you about in the first place.

My final thought: what I've just explained to you is based on science. It's not theory. It *is* how we feel about things and it *is* how we make or don't make purchase decisions. Please don't think it doesn't apply to your patients or that your town is somehow exempt from it.

TALK TO ME AS YOU MOVE THROUGH THE BOOK:

LET ME KNOW YOUR THOUGHTS AND COMMENTS OVER ON TWITTER OR INSTAGRAM:

@THEPAULGOUGH // #ASKPG

COMMON OBJECTIONS TO PHYSICAL THERAPY

My five-year-old son, Harry, tells me he can't put his school clothes on because he doesn't know where they are. That is his excuse. What it *really* means is that the lazy little sod doesn't want to stop watching Power Rangers, get off the couch, and go to his bedroom to look for them. That's what it *really* means.

When someone tells you that the reason they were late is because they were stuck in traffic, that is the excuse. What it *really* means is they didn't leave the house with an appropriate amount of time factored in for excess traffic.

When someone tells you that they didn't have time to read the book you told them about, that is the excuse. What it really means is they prioritized their time elsewhere; they likely valued Facebook and watching Netflix more than your suggested book.

Similarly, when a patient tells you that they can't afford to hire you, that is the excuse. What it *really* means is that they have a cash flow issue. They just don't know how to tell you or expect you to be able to understand.

In most situations, with most patients, the reason they tell you they can't hire you is not actually what they mean. What people say and what they really mean are rarely the same thing. In this chapter, I'm going to explain what the most common objections really mean so you can better handle them.

1. I CAN'T AFFORD IT

This is likely to be the number one excuse you'll hear from patients who tell you they don't want to hire you. But what does it really mean? Well, it means they *do* want to hire you—they just don't have the cash in the bank right now to do so. As I said above, this is a *cash flow issue* and it is important that you understand how it differs from other excuses. It's not that they don't want you, or that they don't see the value, it's that they really don't have the cash at hand to be able to proceed right now.

When the Apple iPhone X came out in 2017, it was priced around $1,000. At the same time, it was reported that something like 64 percent of Americans will never have $1,000 in the bank at any one time in their life. Yet, that didn't stop people from buying the phone. A silly little thing like not having access to the $1,000 needed to buy the phone didn't get in the way of people buying the phone. Someway, somehow, despite not being able to afford it, people bought the iPhone X.

How is that possible? Simple. They flocked to the companies that offered things like payment plans or interest-free loans. Apple and its resellers recognized this "lack of cash flow" issue and came along with an option for people to get access to a phone that they otherwise wouldn't have been able to afford.

And you must do the same. Do anything to make it easier for people to afford to hire you. That doesn't necessarily mean drop your price, it means break the payments up into smaller chunks. It means you might have to find a way to get started with them by offering them a session every other week at first. Then, let them make their way to the full plan of care that they need when they do have the cash at hand.

Either way, to help them, you must first recognize what they're really saying; that is, they just don't have the money at hand to give you right now.

What is more, and what really happened in the case of iPhone X, is that Apple's marketing department did a great job of positioning the product as a must-have item.

Their marketing built up such desire for the product that people were willing to do anything to get it, including use credit cards or take monthly payment options. Even Disney does it. I'm a resident of Florida and when I was purchasing my family's Disney Florida Resident Annual Passes (which cost way more than $1,000), I was given the option of a small down payment and then to pay the rest each month. The smaller monthly payment option is used by all of the top companies on the planet and is how they can charge higher prices for their services.

The lesson is this: having both a smaller monthly payment plan option and a compelling marketing message is going to limit how many times you'll hear this objection. That's because the majority of people in your town will never have access to $1,000 at any one time, simply because they're spending their money faster than they can earn it. They've allocated most of their paycheck to other stuff. It means that they're spending it buying other things like their kids' upcoming birthday or Christmas gifts, a family vacation, a new car, or a TV for the home. Whatever it is, the money they have comes in one day and out the next—if not before.

MEET MY SISTER CLAIRE

My younger sister is a classic example of this. I've never known her to ever have more than $50 in the bank—even on pay day. Yet, she lives an amazing life. She's always off to somewhere exotic like Greece or Spain or Bali, or to a weekend at a spa. If she's not doing that, she's "investing" in a new car or a new item of clothing to wear for another bachelorette weekend she's going on. She's good at earning it, and she's even better at spending it. She never lets the fact that she can't afford it get in the way of buying it.

The thing for you to recognize is that this "I can't afford it" excuse simply means there's a cash flow issue. There's a lag between what they need to spend with you and the next time they'll have that money available to them.

When you hear this, you should *not* be trying to prove value. You should not try convincing them how great you are. Don't even show them case studies or continue talking about your credentials; it doesn't and won't make any difference as there's no money in the bank. What you should be doing is focusing on making it easier for them to pay you in smaller chunks.

Offer payment plans or allow them to take baby steps with you in terms of how much they need to give up before the next time they get paid. Display some empathy and understanding for their situation and give them an option to split the payment over a few months. At the very least, follow up with them so that next month, when the kid's birthday is paid for, the surplus cash they have is cash they can give to you. The *fortune is always in the follow up.*

As I always say, they'll buy into you once they understand that *you* understand their real concerns. Best of all, they'll become a patient for life. In this case, their real issue is cash flow.

2. IT'S TOO EXPENSIVE

"You're just too expensive" is a line I am sure you hear regularly (if you don't, your prices are way too low). But does it *really* mean you're too expensive? Of course it doesn't. It means that they *don't see the value* right now and if you want their commitment, you're going to have to work a little harder to prove that value to them. It could also mean that you're not doing a very good job of showing people how what you do is so different from any other option they've got.

When most owners hear this objection, they falsely assume that it means the person doesn't have the money. It is almost certainly what the staff assumes when they hear this objection. But that isn't the case. If you listen to the words they're using, they're not saying that at all. What they're saying is, "So far I've not seen enough from you to want to give this amount to you."

In this situation, they are screaming for more proof of value.

Now the problem with value is this: it is a concept. It means something different to everyone. What's more, at the beginning of the relationship with a new patient, your value is perceived. It is their *opinion* on the value you might bring to their life in exchange for the time and money they must give you.

It is easy to think that your value is in the clinical skills: the diagnosis, the treatment, or the exercises, etc. To a certain point, it is. However, in the beginning, they can't feel any of that. It means their understanding of your value is derived from their perception of what you'll do for them. The good news for you is their perception is very easily altered.

DON'T GET DEFENSIVE

When you first hear patients say that you're too expensive, it is easy to take it personally, to assume that they think you're trying to rip them off or that you're greedy for charging what you're asking.

Here's my best advice: whatever you do, do not take this personally or to heart and do not get emotional or defensive in any way. Don't try to justify what you're charging. All you have to do is spend more time talking to them about the other people like them you have previously helped.

Remind them of the other people just like them who had similar problems but *did* see the value and got results. Now is the time to bring out your amazing case studies. Now is also the time to connect with them emotionally about the deep-rooted underlying issue that they have. If you do that, they're more likely to want to get started immediately.

If they're telling you that you're too expensive, do not be tempted to instantly drop your price. Simply get them to start talking more about what they want and keep acknowledging that you can achieve that for them. The longer you do that, the more they'll begin to feel comfortable with the prospect of paying your fees.

Remember this: if they're saying "no" because of an uncomfortable feeling, then they'll say "yes" because of the opposite—a comfortable feeling. Make them feel that way and you'll get the "yes" you're looking for.

The ultimate goal of your clinic's sales system is to get them as comfortable as possible, as quickly as possible. That is why three-minute phone calls simply won't do, nor will talking about your credentials or experience. They don't really care. All they want to know is if what you will do for them is worth paying the price you are asking. All they want to know is whether they will have success.

GET YOUR FREE SALES KIT: WWW.PAULGOUGH.COM/SALES-KIT

3. "I NEED TO USE INSURANCE"

Do they really need to use insurance? Or were they just *expecting* to be able to use it? There's a big difference. Sure, they call up and ask about it right away, but why wouldn't they? What else do they know to ask you?

For most people, asking "Do you take my insurance?" is akin to asking a guy or girl in a bar, "Do you come here often?" But does the guy really want to know if the cute girl comes to the bar often? Of course he doesn't. He wants to know significantly more than that, he just doesn't know how to ask anything else.

I hear this one at my clinic all the time. And when people call my clinic and ask if we take their insurance, and we don't, we're very careful about how we answer their question. We *used* to respond with "*Unfortunately* we don't" or "No, *but I can still take you on.*" That was until I realized that both of those responses were doing absolutely nothing to win us a patient.

The problem with the insurance question is simply this: because they lead with the question, you're tricked into thinking that it is the only thing they really want to talk about. You're also thinking that it is the only thing that matters in their decision.

When you respond with "Unfortunately I don't" or "No, but..." it's obvious you're trying to keep the conversation alive. The reality is that you've instantly lost them.

"Unfortunately" and "but" are two words they are used to hearing when the outcome isn't going to be the one they want.

You can try to sell them on a cash pay option, but because they know they're not getting what they came looking for, you're fighting a losing battle. The moment that they hear the word "no," it spooks them. They were hoping for a "yes." They had a follow-up conversation for "yes." But they don't know how to respond to you not taking their insurance. Their only option is to respond with something like, "Okay, thank you" and proceed to put the phone down on you.

Wouldn't it be great if they asked, "Do you have any other options for me to work with you?"

GET YOUR FREE SALES KIT: WWW.PAULGOUGH.COM/SALES-KIT

Wouldn't it be great if they called your clinic and said, "Hello, I love your website, it had some very helpful information on there about how you can solve my specific back problem and I'm hoping to work with you. Could you please tell me how I go about working with you and what types of payments you accept?"

In an ideal world, that's what they would ask. That is what we *want* them to ask, but just because they don't ask it, it doesn't mean you can't answer that question for them.

ASK THE QUESTIONS THEY SHOULD HAVE ASKED

Asking better questions is the key to solving problems in your life—and they're also the gateway to better conversations with patients.

Let me give you an example. If I've taken my two boys out to the park, when we return, Natalie will ask me something like, "Were the boys good?" or "Were they *okay*?" That type of question drives me mad! It's an awful question. What can I say in reply to her? It's either "Yes they were," or, "No, they weren't."

In a very fun way, and to Natalie's complete frustration, I have learned to stop myself from answering this question when she asks me. Instead, I'll often respond with something like, "I think what you wanted to know was did we have fun?" or "What did we get up to without you?" Of course, she hates me for doing this, and after smiling in a way that confirms that she does, she then proceeds to listen and enjoy hearing all about the *wonderful* experiences her children have just had.

Because I answered the question she should have asked, she got a much better response. She got a much better outcome. I added value to her life.

The point? This is what you need to do with patients. If you answer the insurance question with "yes" or "no," you're doing them a disservice. They're going to miss out on knowing about all of the other ways in which you could still help them and add value to their life—despite not taking their insurance. Remember that most people do not fully understand their health insurance; they have a false belief that everything will be covered by their insurance and need to be educated on insurance in general. You can do that for them if you ask them a question that is something like, "Is using insurance the only thing that matters to you when you decide which physical therapist you will choose, or are you concerned more about value?"

If you ask the question they should have asked, you might help them to understand that what you're offering, although not covered by insurance, might offer them more value than actually using insurance.

4. "I DON'T HAVE TIME"

Really? They don't have time? Of course they do. They just don't want to give up time somewhere else in their life. If they're telling you that they don't have the time, it really means they don't think the juice is going to be worth the squeeze.

I realized a long time ago that the time excuse has nothing to do with the actual availability of time. Instead, it has everything to do with how they value time. The issue here is a *lack* of certainty. It is a lack of certainty in the outcome they're going to get for the time they're going to have to give up.

When you think about this one, what they are really saying is this: "I'm not going to make adjustments to my plans to fit this in if I am *not sure* it is even going to work for me." And why would they? Why would anyone make changes to their day for something that they perceive isn't certain?

As we discussed in the previous chapter on cognitive dissonance, physical therapy is an uncertain outcome and what they perceive matters more than what you or I believe to be truth. And, if you can't make them feel certain or alter their perception, then they'll always side with spending an hour on Facebook rather than with you.

You'll often see the same people who tell you that they "don't have time for physical therapy" sit in a hair salon spending hundreds of dollars or goofing off on the golf course spending a lot of money to do so.

The same lady who tells you she can't get someone to look after her kids—and therefore doesn't have time to come for physical therapy—will nearly always find someone to look after the kids when it comes to getting hair and nails done.

How do I know? Because it happens in my own house every month. Natalie is forever telling me how busy she is and that "she doesn't have time" to do things anymore since we've had kids. Yet, she never seems to miss *that* appointment with the girl who does her hair and nails. She'll call in a favor from *any* family member or friend to look after the kids while she goes to the nail salon. Would she do it for physical therapy if she had a bad back? I'm not so sure.

So why does she move heaven and earth to make the hair appointment happen? It's because there is 100 percent certainty in the outcome she gets when she goes there.

She knows for an absolute fact that when she arrives at the hair or nail salon, she walks out 60 minutes later looking and feeling fabulous. She knows people will notice the difference in how she looks (except me) and they'll comment on it (except me). In this situation, she is certain in the outcome she is going to get and therefore she will do whatever it takes to make the appointment happen. Including finding someone to watch the kids.

My point? It's not a time thing, it's how certain they are about how they are going to feel about giving up their time and what the reward will be if they do. It's always been this way and always will be this way.

Please don't take any of this the wrong way—I'm just pointing out *not-so obvious* facts. This is the fundamental law of how humans behave. The point I am bringing to your attention is that your patients are not that busy. No one is. The President of the United States finds more time to play golf than your patients need to give up to come and see you.

Your patients are making a decision with their time based upon the certainty—or the lack of it—that they perceive in you. How much of their time you get is directly proportional to how much certainty you offer. If they feel it from you, they'll prioritize you. If they don't, they won't, and you'll hear this excuse constantly. If they're not ringing their long-lost cousin or the friend who lives around the corner to look after the kids so they can come see you, it's because they don't believe it's worth it. When the outcome is certain, people find time.

GET YOUR FREE SALES KIT: WWW.PAULGOUGH.COM/SALES-KIT

5. "I'LL WAIT A LITTLE LONGER AND SEE HOW IT GOES

Most patients forget or at the very least are unsure of how long they've actually been suffering with their problem. Why not remind them? Simply point out that what they're about to do (wait for more time) is actually what they've already tried. Oh, and of course don't forget to point out that *it hasn't worked.*

If they've called you, it's a good sign that they're fed up with their problem. Unless they want a sick note for a day off work, people don't call the doctor when they're feeling great. No, they usually call the doctor days after their symptoms started, or, to be more precise, when whatever they've tried so far hasn't worked.

It's the same with physical therapy. You're unlikely to be their first attempt to correct their problem; it could be months or even years after having tried other things that they find their way to you.

I've experienced a number of occasions where a patient has arrived for an initial consultation and has forgotten just how long they've been suffering. At first, they'll say it's "only been a couple of weeks" and yet, a session or two later, when they really feel comfortable with me, they'll let it slip that the "two-week-old" knee problem actually started some eighteen months ago.

"Now that I think about it, I've had this problem since..." is the typical line I hear regularly.

Given that most people can't remember what they did last night, it's safe to assume that they won't always be wholly accurate at remembering precisely when their pain started.

Your job is to ask the right questions to confirm precisely when it did start—and remind them of that. Simply ask them questions that take them back to what life was like *before* their knee problem started, however long ago it was. We want patients to understand for themselves that waiting for more time isn't going to help them. When that happens, you're going to get their buy-in. People are irrational, they're easily confused, but they're *not* stupid.

GET YOUR FREE SALES KIT: WWW.PAULGOUGH.COM/SALES-KIT

Remind them that time is something that they've already tried and they're less likely to want to give it any more time. The definition of insanity is doing the same thing every day and expecting a different result. Your patients are not insane. They are just forgetful.

DO THEY KNOW THE IMPLICATIONS OF WAITING?

Most of the time, patients have no understanding of the implications of leaving it a little longer. They've lost sight of the consequences of leaving it to the mercy of yet more time. As you and I both know, when it comes to knee or back problems, time does nothing but make them worse and take longer to heal. It's your job to remind them of that.

If I go to the dentist with a little sensitivity or pain, I hope that my dentist will point out that I do indeed have a small cavity and remind me that there is no such thing as "waiting." Once I have decay, it will only continue to get worse. And if I had been waiting for long enough already with a little discomfort, she wouldn't be doing her job if she let me keep waiting and hoping that the cavity would go away.

Here's an interesting question: when faced with that type of situation, what would you hope your dentist does for you? How do you hope that your dentist treats you?

a) Politely and respectfully reminds you of the consequences of delaying the proper course of treatment.

Or

b) Ignore having the conversation with you, just in case you accuse him of selling to you.

I know I would prefer the former, and I am sure you would too. Why not just do for your patients as you would like to be done to you? Focus on being respected—not liked.

GET YOUR FREE SALES KIT: WWW.PAULGOUGH.COM/SALES-KIT

6. "IT WON'T WORK FOR ME"

Some people will never play the lottery because they believe they're so unlucky that they're never going to win. Some people believe that they're so unlucky in love that there is no point in even creating an online dating account. They know online dating works for others, but because "it's them," it will never work. The same person knows that Oprah's new diet really does work, but not for people like them with "big bones" inherited from their grandmother. As such, they rule themselves out from even trying it.

This is real life for many people. They carry their same self-limiting beliefs into everything that they do. That includes how they view physical therapy.

There are a lot of people out there who, no matter how good you are, or even how good your reviews say you are, will never feel like they can hire you. That is simply because they doubt it will ever work for someone like them. Even though they call you, they still have major doubts that physical therapy can work *for them*. They have hope—but their doubts always win.

This a huge certainty issue (or lack thereof!) and you cannot beat it by talking about credentials or better treatment techniques.

No, to beat this type of objection you must speak directly to it. Before that, you must first recognize it. The clues will be in their subjective history. They'll tell you that they've tried many things before getting to you and they'll be negative about almost everything—including their visit with you.

The irony is that although they might think it won't work for them, they're still there talking to you. And that is something you must remind them of. Remind them of the fact that if they're calling you, they *do* believe that something can be done.

It's most likely that they're just nervous as they get to the point of having to commit. That nervousness created a seed of doubt that caused them to forget that they *do* think something can be done. Otherwise, why would they call you? You wouldn't ask for a drink if you weren't thirsty, and nor would they ask for help if they didn't think they could be helped.

My tip for you is to not shy away from their obvious doubts. Don't turn a blind eye to them in the hope they will go away. I encourage you to be open with them and talk candidly about the fact that you understand that people are a little concerned that physical therapy might not work for them. Remember, it's only when *they understand* that *you understand them* that they buy from you.

I'd go so far as to encourage you to be upfront about the fact that it may not work for them. Display empathy, but at the same time be certain in the way that you tell them it might not work for them.

Be kind, be caring, and be compassionate—but be firm doing it. It is more about how you say it than what you say. Get them believing in *you* (the person) as that is way more important than them believing in the outcome. If you try to tell them you're 100 percent certain that you can solve their issue, and they've already tried 17 different things before getting to you, there's going to be a disconnect and they'll stall over their decision.

WHAT ARE THE ALTERNATIVES?

Another thing you could do is ask what other alternatives they are considering. If they are reminded that the choice they have is years of pain or giving you a try and getting even just 20 percent better, it is easier for them to rationalize that and start to make the decision to hire you.

As always, what they want is for you to be direct and honest, acknowledging that you understand what they're feeling. When the patient begins to realize that you understand how they are really feeling, they come to their own conclusion that you are different from anyone else. That is when trust starts to be built. That is when they want to hire you no matter what you charge. That is the key to all success with true sales.

It is also at this point that something really magical happens—they start to buy into you the person (not the therapist).

When you are upfront and honest about what is possible for them, about the fact that you may only be able to make slight improvements in their health, all of a sudden they're not buying physical therapy or any

GET YOUR FREE SALES KIT: WWW.PAULGOUGH.COM/SALES-KIT

type of treatment—they're buying *you* and your ability to understand them. You'll likely be the very first person in their history of this problem to be brutally honest with them and face up to the fact that yes, it might not work—but it's better to try something than suffer and never know.

What is more, they can't or won't be left feeling disappointed at the other end if you do this. And that is important. Many people fear the disappointment of making yet another mistake more than they do losing their money. If you're confident, honest, and upfront at the start about what is possible and probable, they can't suffer yet another disappointment if it doesn't work out. They feel better about that already. Essentially, you are under promising to win their trust and you're going to *overdeliver* when you get it.

The key point here is that you're only going to do this with someone who doesn't think it will work for them. You're not under promising everyone or telling every patient that you might not be able to help them, only the ones who have a list as long as their arm of prior things they've tried that didn't work. They're going to be attracted to your brutal honesty and, because of that, they're more likely to say "yes" to you.

By the way, don't be surprised how many people are waiting for you to be brutally honest with them. Don't think that you have to tell everyone you can get them 100 percent better. Don't overpromise what you can do. If you do, they'll use it as an excuse to not proceed. They'll tell themselves that you're just like everyone else who has already let them down.

Being successful in this situation requires an acknowledgement of their doubts and fears and recognizing that they have been let down in the past. They need to know that you understand why they currently feel the way they do. When you do this, you are now showing more compassion and empathy than this person has ever likely felt in the past—and *that* is why they'll choose to hire you.

7. "IT'S TOO FAR TO TRAVEL"

No it isn't. They just don't think you're any different from the physical therapist who is close to their house or office. Harsh, but true. Nothing is ever too far to travel for; there is, however, a lack of motivation to do so.

In Chapter 2, I spoke about preeminence and a lack it being the root cause of a lot of selling and conversion issues in physical therapy. "It is too far to travel" is a classic symptom—the effect.

If you think that no one will travel twenty-five miles to see you, how do you explain the thousands of patients who are flying across the country (and even into different countries) to access health care providers that they want to see? You might be saying to yourself "Oh, but they won't do that for physical therapy," I would agree. And this is my point. They will not travel twenty-five miles to see another physical therapist—not when there's one right on their doorstep.

In the same way that people will not pay more for the same thing that they believe they can get cheaper, nor will they travel an hour to access the same thing that is right by their house. That is why you have to use preeminence and positioning to make sure that you don't look or feel like any option they've got that is closer to them.

If you position yourself as an expert, able to solve the specific problem that they have, they will come and see you, just like people will get on flights and travel cross country. In the same way they won't pay more to get the same thing, nor will they want to see the generalist if they have the choice of the specialist.

The key is to use your marketing to change their perception of what you do so that you're no longer just a physical therapist. Instead, you're talking to them about a specific problem that they have and how you know precisely how to solve it. If people are getting on a plane to travel across the country, it's because their perception is that they are traveling to see the one person who is able to solve their specific problem. Marketing does that for you.

Use your marketing to help them differentiate between you and every other option so that they do want to go through rush hour traffic and into a different town to come and see you. The stronger your marketing message, the easier is it for them to distinguish why you're different and why they should incur that inconvenience.

You could also tell stories of other people who have visited you who travelled even farther than the person you're speaking to. Social proof is incredibly powerful in the sales process. If they hear the story of the guy or girl who travelled two hours every day to get to you for four weeks, it

GET YOUR FREE SALES KIT: WWW.PAULGOUGH.COM/SALES-KIT

makes their thirty-minute trip across town seem like a stroll in the park on a sunny day.

Ok, so there are the seven common objections you should be aware of. If you want the exact scripts and templates I use to overcome these objections, you should enroll in my instant access program: "Effortless Selling System: Double Front Desk And Treatment Conversions in Just 48 Hours." It is an online program that comes complete with a physical binder sent to you in the mail within a few days of enrolling. Everything you need is available to you instantly and you can start overcoming these objections with ease starting today. Get the program here: **www.PatientConversionSystem.com/book.**

TALK TO ME AS YOU MOVE THROUGH THE BOOK:

LET ME KNOW YOUR THOUGHTS AND COMMENTS OVER ON TWITTER OR INSTAGRAM:

@THEPAULGOUGH // #ASKPG

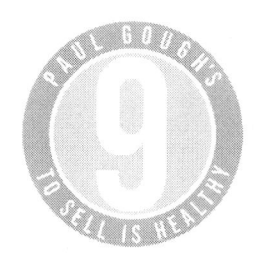

HOW TO INFLUENCE WITH INTEGRITY – THE FIVE STEPS TO "EFFORTLESS SELLING"

Now that you know what the objections are, and what they really mean, let's walk through a process that I've developed that'll help you to *influence your patients with integrity*.

So far in the book, we have covered many of the foundational principles and behavioral science behind selling physical therapy services using the process I've developed and termed, "EFFORTLESS SELLING."

In this chapter, we're going to bring many of those into a step-by-step process that you can follow from now on. There are five steps to the Effortless Selling process, and you should follow each one in the order that you're about to discover them.

Part 1: Build Rapport

Part 2: Value Alignment

Part 3: Match Benefits to Their Specific Problem

Part 4: Anticipate Their Objections

Part 5: Ask If They are Happy to Proceed

Let's start with:

PART 1: BUILD RAPPORT

Here's how most consultations with a physical therapist begin:

"So, Dr. Smith has referred you for knee pain. What's been going on?"

And a receptionist might start with:

"What is your insurance?"

These two types of conversations are very easy to have at the beginning. The problem is that when you go straight to this type of thing, you miss a fundamental aspect of the sales process: building rapport.

People buy from people. And if you move straight to the type of conversation you would expect between a patient and clinician, then there's been no rapport built between two human beings.

Look back at all of the people who have said yes to you in the last twelve months. I bet that they mostly have one thing in common: you spent more time *getting to know them as a person* before the conversation about their pain or their insurance started.

Receptionists are often guilty of this primarily because they're so time starved. The phone rings with an inquiry from a patient and it's a case of getting off the phone as fast as possible because someone else is in the waiting room or on the other line. It means the entire conversation is about the necessaries: the cost, the location, the parking, hours, the therapist, and insurance. All of this is done in three minutes flat and there's little if any time that allows for building rapport.

Most clinic owners can't afford the luxury of allocating time to building rapport. As a result, they stay stuck. The reality is they're not making enough money to bring in a second receptionist to do this simply because the first one doesn't have time to do it right.

If you can't afford to do the things that you need to do to make the money you want, how do you expect to grow?

Something else to consider is that just because patients arrive, it doesn't mean they're fully committed. Just because they're on your schedule, it doesn't mean they're as invested in your service as they would be if you build rapport with them. Don't confuse arrival with commitment.

People often make very small commitments with people they don't have rapport with. If you keep hearing patients decline a plan of care and only book out one or two sessions, it is likely that rapport is missing. Building rapport means they'll not only make a bigger commitment with you, but that they'll spend more with you as well.

Simply put, spending some time getting to know the person before you consider them a client or patient is something that you and your front desk people must do. No one buys anything of significant value from someone that they don't get along with or feel connected to. If they do not connect with you, that dissonance that I spoke about earlier in the book builds and the result is that they feel uncomfortable about you. This is what they end up saying no to—not your skills or your prices.

CLINICIANS FRESH OUT OF SCHOOL

I've seen this in full effect from both sides of the rapport spectrum. On one hand, I've employed very skilled practitioners who struggle with getting people to say yes. Equally, I've seen therapists fresh out of school (with fewer clinical skills) have zero problems with conversions.

What makes the difference is often rapport.

Highly skilled practitioners often want to go straight to the conversation that they're comfortable with: the clinical one. It means they struggle to connect with patients emotionally. As a result, patients say "no" and it's simply because they do not feel comfortable. It happens when there's too much emphasis on the clinical aspect of what you do for people and not enough on the people aspect. EQ is way more important than IQ.

That is why whenever I look to recruit new therapists for my practice, I am looking for this above everything else. I care less about where they went to school and more about how easy it is to build rapport with them.

I have no doubt you do this in your own life too. You will likely visit places primarily because of the rapport that you have with the people who run the establishment. I know I do. That is the situation that you want to be in. You want people buying into you and your people and how you make them feel as human beings, not just as patients. They'll only do that if you take the time to build some kind of person-to-person rapport with them before you talk about what they need as a patient.

THE POWER OF RAPPORT IN ACTION

I once did a talk in Montreal, Canada, for one of the biggest physical therapy franchises in the country. There was something like 27 clinics that made up the group. The day before my talk, I was taken to visit some of the clinics to see the staff in action. As the story goes, I walked into one clinic and one particular therapist made a point of coming over to talk to me. He started by asking where I was from and so I told him— England.

England is a place known throughout the world for soccer, and this guy knew immediately to strike up a conversation with me about it. We spoke for five minutes or so about our favorite teams. I told him I supported Liverpool and he told me he supported Manchester United. I told him my favorite player was Steven Gerrard and he told me his was Wayne Rooney (two very big players in UK soccer). On and on this conversation went.

What was he doing? That is right, he was building rapport with me.

After the conversation, I watched him go back to his patients and I saw him do exactly the same thing with them. He spoke to the *person* at length before he got to their need to be considered a patient.

This is something I have drummed into the staff of my own clinic for years. There's not just a patient sitting in front of you, there's a person— a person who does not want to be defined or labeled for having a swollen knee. There's a person who has a favorite soccer team, grandchildren, hobbies, and interests. You must talk about these things before you ask about their knee pain. This is precisely what the therapist in this story was doing.

The next day, when I was on stage speaking to all of the physical therapists in the franchise, I commented on my experience with the therapist in question. I told the room how impressed I was. More, I made a bold statement that based solely upon my experience with the therapist the day before, I'd be happy to wager a lot of money that he was one of the highest-producing therapists in the entire franchise. I was certain that this guy would be one of the therapists in this room with the highest number of visits against his name per new patients he sees.

Turns out I was wrong. He wasn't one of the highest—he was *the* highest. And the reason was he had the most basic of things covered in the sales process—the ability to strike up rapport with patients. He had an *effortless* ability to sell to people, much as I explained earlier in the book.

I hadn't seen this guy in action as a clinician. I had no clue how experienced he was or what skills he even had. However, I knew that he knew how to build rapport with people as well as anyone I've ever seen. It's for that reason that so many people wanted to get on his schedule. He was selling them a feeling that others couldn't. He was changing the meaning of what people were paying for. He was doing all of the things I've spoken about so far in this book.

In your clinic right now, this is either happening or it's not. And if it isn't, you must make a shift to spending more time getting to know more about people—no matter how long it takes.

I can say confidently, from years of doing this, that the longer you spend in the rapport-building phase, not only will your conversions increase, but so too the amount of money they will spend with you. There's a direct correlation between the time spent getting to know them before they have to spend money with you and how much money they go on to spend with you after. Said differently, the more you spend with them (time), the more they spend with you (money).

PART 2: VALUE ALIGNMENT

The second part of the system is about aligning value—the value that you bring and the value that they want. I've often heard it said that you have to show them the value of what you do if you want them to buy from you. It sounds great in theory, but it can only work if you actually know what they really value. That is why you need to ask them the right questions.

It's very unlikely that what they value is what you think they value. That is the number one reason for a disconnect between therapist and patient. You think that they should value an increase in their ankle

ROM— and yet what they really value is the ability to walk along the beach without their ankle hurting. The two are not the same.

Most therapists erroneously believe that value is found in providing one-on-one attention or being superior at "dry needling" or some exercise fad that is proven to ease back pain. Those things are important, but they're just *features* that go into providing the benefit and ultimately the value that the patient is looking for (i.e., walking along the beach pain free).

At first glance, none of us can ever know what the patient really values. That's why it's important to ask them the right questions.

You'll get the best answers if you move away from the stereotypical clinical questions such as, "On a scale of one to ten, how bad is your pain?" and instead start asking things like, "If I could solve this problem for you, what value would it bring to your life?"

Notice how I'm asking *them* what value looks like. When I know this, it changes the conversation and ultimately the outcome of that conversation. It's then much easier to match up what I can do for them with what they want.

The questions that we have been trained to ask in the subjective phase of our initial assessments are primarily for the benefit of the insurance company or efficiently completing the EMR. Neither is very helpful in finding out what they will value. The problem is they do not in any way assist someone who is nervous or skeptical about beginning this journey with you to discriminate in your favor and hire you. All of your typical initial consultation questions elicit a logical response. Yet, if you want people to buy from you, they're more likely to do so when they're emotional.

SPENDING MORE THAN WAS PLANNED

As I write this section of the book, it is two days after Christmas Day and people have most likely spent hundreds if not thousands more on Christmas presents than they initially budgeted. Why is that? Well, it's because Christmas is *the* most emotional time of the year. The budget tends to fly out the window when they are actually in the store shopping, imagining the look of joy on their loved ones' faces when they open the gift.

Value-based questions move people to an emotional state where they like to do their buying—and more of it. With that in mind, here are two questions that you could ask your patients that would lead you into a more emotional conversation:

1. "How long have you suffered and what has held you back from coming to see me up until now?"

2. "Why did you feel like that for so long?"

Ask those two questions and then shut up! Put your hand over your mouth if you have to—but once you've asked them, you must go quiet. Even if they go quiet for two or three seconds, it just means they're thinking. The best questions have the longest silences. You've asked them two questions that no one ever has before and now they're thinking. You're about to get to the heart of the real problem that is holding them back. When you know what it is, you can talk about the real problem until it's not a problem any longer.

> **There are more questions like this when you register your book and collect your complimentary Sales Tool Kit.**
> **Do that here: www.paulgough.com/sales-kit**

PART 3: MATCH BENEFITS TO THEIR SPECIFIC PROBLEM

By and large, most people's sales problems are caused by a lack of specificity in what they're selling. Physical therapy is perceived as a general solution to any number of problems. And that is the problem. Physical therapy can be used for any number of things; therefore, it is easy for it to end up getting used for very few. There's a good reason very few generalists ever get rich.

There's always been "riches in niches," but now, more than ever, that saying is true. The whole thing is made worse by the fact that new clinics are opening regularly, and that means the number of people selling a general solution is increasing.

GET YOUR FREE SALES KIT: WWW.PAULGOUGH.COM/SALES-KIT

The generalized public perception is that *all* physical therapists sell the same thing: exercises and maybe some type of massage, perhaps? The result is a race to the bottom, as consumers have no option but to choose based on price—the cheapest.

The key to avoiding the race to the bottom is to specialize, to provide a highly specific solution to a highly specific problem. When you do, they are not just more likely to say "yes," they will do so *at higher prices too*.

This part of the five-step process is about matching up the benefits of your service with their specific problem. And if you follow this process, it's really easy to do. The previous step was about finding out what they value. If you ask them the right questions, then they will tell you what they value. From then on, it is easy to match up what you do in relation to what they want. They'll pay for what they want. They won't pay for what the insurance company or your EMR wants, so don't follow their line of questioning. You'll end up asking questions that lead to conversations about pain relief or restoration of function. It's something that you do, but not the best thing you can do for them. And it certainly is not what they'll pay you the most money for.

Asking this type of question is better:

"What value would it bring to your life in the next three weeks if I could solve this problem for you?"

It might be that the patient replies with something like they would, "Finally be able to go hiking without having to worry about excruciating back pain the next day." And when they do, you can then start to talk to them about how *that* is precisely what you do.

Pain relief and function will be taken care of, but there's a bigger, higher purpose that they're hiring you for. There's a bigger outcome that they're happy to pay more for.

Once you know what they really want, as discussed earlier in the book, the easiest way to sell them on getting their outcome is to tell a story. Ideally, tell a story of another patient that you've treated recently who received that exact outcome. Talk to them about someone with similar values that you have helped get the desired result they're dreaming of right now. You might say something like:

GET YOUR FREE SALES KIT: WWW.PAULGOUGH.COM/SALES-KIT

"I hear this story all the time. In fact, just recently I helped a lady in her mid-fifties who had suffered with low back pain that had kept her from hiking with friends for six months. She was finally able to make it to the top of her favorite mountain. In fact, she just shared with me a picture of her and her husband at the top enjoying the view together."

In that instant, and simply by recalling a story of a similar patient who wanted a similar outcome, I've communicated with this person that I understand their specific problem. Second, I've demonstrated that I can provide a specific solution to a very specific problem.

Do this, and while your competition are focused primarily on the low back pain and improving this person's pain score, you're talking about getting this patient back to hiking and great conversations with friends while they walk—without the frustration of nagging back pain getting in the way.

BECOME AN OVERNIGHT SPECIALIST WITHOUT SPENDING THOUSANDS ON CEUS

Becoming a specialist can happen really fast. It is also much easier than having to spend tens of thousands of dollars to get more continuing education or CEUs in a specific area of physical therapy. You don't need to have dozens of certificates hanging from the wall to be a specialist in helping a lady in her mid-fifties to get back to hiking. You just need to communicate the fact that you've done it many times before.

It's not about becoming a specialist in a clinical skill set; it's about becoming what I call a *patient-focused specialist*. It's about becoming the specialist they need you to be. It's about asking the patient what they want to achieve and then becoming a specialist in the thing that they tell you they want to achieve. Becoming a specialist in achieving things is a lot more powerful than being a specialist in doing things (such as certain treatment techniques.)

With all of this in mind, it would be a good idea for you to start documenting some common stories that you might need to relay to future patients. Keeping a notebook of all your amazing success stories that are relevant to your perfect patient allows you to effortlessly sell through stories. I have all of my front desk team pay extra attention to the patients who come in and then later write down the stories they tell us.

GET YOUR FREE SALES KIT: WWW.PAULGOUGH.COM/SALES-KIT

We want to be able to recall and tell their story to the next patient who calls us with a similar situation.

PART 4: ANTICIPATE THEIR OBJECTIONS

Once you've built rapport, you've asked your value-aligning questions, and you've told them a story that matches up with what they are hoping to achieve, the next thing you must do is anticipate objections.

Just because the patient hasn't expressed an objection or a concern, do not assume that there isn't one. Even if they say there isn't one, it is very likely that objections will pop up later. It's when the patient returns home that doubts or questions crop up and you want to have answered them before then.

The very worst thing you can do at this point is to assume that everything is going well; that because you told the story that matched up to their benefits, they're 100 percent bought into hiring you. They might be. But it's safer to assume they're not.

If patients do not raise any questions or objections, I worry that they either do not understand the process, are agreeing with me to avoid confrontation, or they're not feeling comfortable enough to say "no." At any rate, it is not good. That is why at this point, if they have not raised an objection, you must ask if they have one.

How do you do it? Simply ask them.

Say something like, "At this point, most people have questions that they want answered before they leave. What questions do you have for me?"

Note that I did not ask "Do you have questions for me?" That is because they will most likely say "no." Asking them *what questions* forces them to think of one. The quality of the question changes the quality of the answer.

GET YOUR FREE SALES KIT: WWW.PAULGOUGH.COM/SALES-KIT

PART 5: ASK IF THEY ARE HAPPY TO PROCEED

What is the easiest way to lose weight? It is to put down the damn fork! What is the easiest and fastest way to boost sales? Simply ask, "Are you ready to proceed and book the appointment?" Like putting down the fork, it is so simple, yet most people can't bring themselves around to doing it, or they forget!

When you ask, only one of two things can happen. If they say "yes," great, job well done!

If they say "no," that is also great. You're about to find out what the objection was that you so far have not covered for them. There's no way you can lose, and yet this is the bit that most people dread or fear.

I appreciate that the silence that follows right after you ask is not easy, but the more you do it, the more comfortable you get with it. The key to this step in the process is to not be connected to the outcome. From now on, you can't care whether it is a "yes" or a "no."

I look at it this way: I want it to be a "yes" for their sake, not mine. If it is a "yes," it is just another part of my day. If it is a "no," it is just another part of my day. There's nothing to celebrate if a patient says "yes," there's nothing to be down about if they say "no." It's a flatline all the way.

If a patient says "yes," I like to think that they are the ones who stand to gain more than me. I get a lot of pleasure from helping, but they get their life changed. If they say "no," sadly, it's them who stands to miss out most. It's a mindset thing that makes you immune from rejection. I want to help them for their sake, but whatever they say, I am not downhearted. I am going home to two beautiful children who love me regardless of whether a patient says "yes" *or* "no."

Never forget that you've got something like that in your life. Whether it is family or friends, you've got people who love and respect you for who you are, not what you do (physical therapy). The former is way more important and is what you will be defined by in the end. Your self-worth and future happiness do not hang on whether a stranger with back pain says "yes" or "no" to you.

GET YOUR FREE SALES KIT: WWW.PAULGOUGH.COM/SALES-KIT

If you hear "no," it just means that they didn't understand your value. It doesn't mean you have no value. Big difference.

HOW TO ASK FOR THE APPOINTMENT

When it comes to the asking, I prefer to give the patient an option. I'll often say something like, "I can do tomorrow at 10 a.m. or Friday at 3:30 p.m. Which one works best for you?" Always give the patient a choice. If they say "no" to both, great, ask them to tell you what time they would prefer.

If they say, "I'm not sure," guess what is there? An objection that you have not covered. The elephant is still in the room and it's getting in the way of the "yes" you both need to hear.

At this point, you should go back and ask them, "What is it that is holding you back?" and then shut up for a few seconds to let them speak.

You'll most likely get one of the excuses that I outlined earlier in the book, but remember that it all goes back to trust—or a lack of it. If they're still saying "no," you haven't earned enough of it yet. But at least you know and you're not living in the perpetual state of helplessness, always thinking that you're so unlucky to get a call from everyone in your town with no money or time.

So, there you have the five steps that bring all of the major principles of this book together. Next, we're going to look at how to raise your prices —without the gut-wrenching, stomach-churning, sickening feeling you get even just thinking about doing it. Come with me to the next chapter and I'll help you get a raise the instant you put down this book.

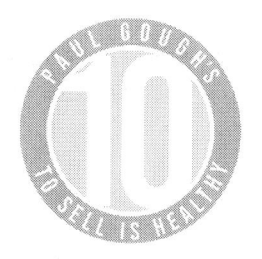

GIVE YOURSELF A RAISE – EFFECTIVE TODAY

I believe that the best thing about being a business owner is that, unlike working for a mill-like physical therapy clinic, you decide when you get a raise. You get to choose when you want an extra thousand dollars in your bank every month.

The problem for many physical therapists is that they'll never exercise that liberty. They're just not that comfortable making their own life easier. They choose to keep their prices low in order to help more people and at the same time bind themselves to a lifetime of struggle where money is scarce and stress is high.

I wonder just how many therapists reading this have spent their entire careers worrying one minute about being judged for what they charge and the next minute hoping for their financial circumstances to change?

Externally, they'll tell you they don't want to charge higher prices because they want to help people. However, privately, they wonder what the point of being in business actually is because there's nothing to show for it—there's never any money in the bank. Fulfillment is important, but let me remind you that it doesn't send your kids to good schools or pay the mortgage.

If this is happening to you, is the problem that you don't want to charge higher prices because you want to help as many people as possible, or is the problem that you're worried about being judged?

From the way I see it, from the thousands of clinic owners I've worked with around the world, I think it is the latter. Most physical therapists are living in a perpetual state of fear over being judged and *that* is the real reason they don't dare raise their prices to a standard that is appropriate for the impact they make.

Can you relate?

HEALING FALSE BELIEFS ABOUT MONEY

It's easy to say that you have issues with money. It's easy to say you are working on "healing some false beliefs" about money and your own self-worth. That's fine as long as they *are* false beliefs about money and not something you're hiding behind.

What do I mean by that? Well, I put it to you that if you've been trying to fix either of those two things (false belief about money and self-worth) for any period of time and you so far haven't, then you're trying to fix the wrong problem. The real issue is yet to be tackled. You're fixing a hamstring strain when the problem is the sciatic nerve.

It's very likely that the real root cause about why you can't raise your rates is the *chronic fear of being judged and rejected*. Those two are nearly always the primary issues when it comes to money and self-worth. They're also the silent killer of success in most areas of life.

This issue of having false beliefs about money and self-worth is not exclusive to a healthcare profession, either. Almost every business owner, in every profession, has this issue. That is because deep down we're all the same. We're all born with a brain that has a primary function of survival and it requires you to feel like you're loved and liked in order to survive.

The problem for most is they never stop and realize that they are *already* loved and liked by the people who actually matter. Wanting to be loved and liked by customers of a private enterprise (the patients of your business) is completely unnecessary and mainly driven by ego.

It took me fourteen years of being an adult to realize that I'd suffered from this problem and from the moment it was pointed out to me, it was obvious that I was playing a zero-sum game. It was also liberating in the way that I looked at life and the things I was doing.

I'm serious when I say I spent the first fourteen years of my adult life thinking that people liking me would increase my self-worth. I falsely assumed that more people liking me (or saying good things about me as a physical therapist) meant that I would be happier and more fulfilled. The reverse was true. It became a constant charade.

It was only when I realized that I felt like I needed to be liked because I lacked love elsewhere in my life that I was able to make a change that set me free.

I'll make a sweeping generalization when I say that most people's incessant need to be liked comes from a lack of love that is missing somewhere else in their life. It's usually missing from a parent and it causes you to feel perpetually insecure. You don't know it, but the only way you know how to cover over that insecurity is to try to be liked by as many people as possible. Including patients.

That was my real problem – is something similar happening to you?

These days I couldn't care less how many likes I get on Facebook or how many people want to say good things about me; I don't care if people book appointments at my clinic or buy my programs or products. I never check review sites for my books or podcasts. I'm respectful and grateful for all these things, but I don't need them to feel good. In the grand scheme of what I want from my life, they're irrelevant.

When I am on my deathbed, I certainly will not be looking on Amazon at the reviews for my books and I will not be looking in my patient database to see how many names I collected. Those things will not define my success or the meaning of my life.

I will, however, be looking into the eyes of my children and before I close mine I will make sure that they never feel the lack of love that I did, the lack of love that caused years of unnecessary angst and feeling like I needed a lot of people to like me in order to feel good about myself. What matters is not how many people love or like you, only that the ones who matter do.

If you take nothing else from me, I hope it is this. Nothing would *thrill* me more than to know that more people are living with less fear and doubt. These can prevent you from living with the confidence and certainty you could have. I hope that if we ever meet in person, you will

GET YOUR FREE SALES KIT: WWW.PAULGOUGH.COM/SALES-KIT

walk up to me with a swagger and confidence *in yourself* that make people wish that they had some of what you've got.

When they ask how you got it, tell them you finally realized that most of the crap you used to worry about was unnecessary… that most of the people you thought you needed to like you were actually irrelevant and that instead of needing approval from patients, you focused on being *respected* by patients. What's more, you focused back in on the love and adoration you already get from the small number of people to whom you are already a hero.

Don't change who you are or give up on who you could be for the sake of pleasing people who will never be pleased. The people who really matter are the *only* ones who matter. Everyone else can either go f**k themselves or agree to play your game. From now on, you don't care which one. And by the way, you're doing this *for* them—not *to* them.

When you take this level of self-belief into all of your situations, especially with patients, watch your conversions soar. Best—the irony about living like this is that more people will like you and want to be around you. Far from being fearful of you, they're attracted to you. It's like I said earlier in this book, people are attracted to someone that they perceive to have something they lack. What is it that they lack? It's that same confidence in themselves that you lacked *before* you picked up this book.

BEYOND EMOTIONAL AWKWARDNESS

Before we finish this book together, I'm keen to help you give yourself a raise. To do that—to raise your rates to the level they should be at—you're going to have to get comfortable and learn to charge people appropriately for what you do.

You've got to go beyond the *emotional awkwardness* about asking for a plastic thing (credit card) or a piece of green colored paper with a picture of a president on it (dollar bills) in exchange for your services. After all, that is all that is happening when you ask for money.

It starts with you ceasing lowering your fees because you think you're taking food off their table if you don't.

How many times have you helped a patient and then at the end said something like, "It's usually $100, but for you I'll do it for $75"? We have all done it at some time or other. And doesn't it feel nice at the time when you do? It might feel good at the time, but it's not nearly as good or pleasurable as being able to tell your wife or husband that you can *finally* pay the mortgage this month or go on vacation. Wouldn't you agree?

Never forget that your business and all of the activity it produces must serve the owner. The dog must wag the tail. If not, the energy you expend on *just scraping by* robs you of your positivity and creativity. And those are two vital things required of you if your clinic is to grow and serve more people.

The cruel irony for many healthcare professionals is that they want to help as many people as they can; they think that if they keep prices low, then they can do that. Sounds great in theory. But tell that to the arthritic joints in your hands that caused you to stop treating ten years earlier than you would have liked.

Far from being the gateway to helping more people, an inability to charge money for what you do is going to be the number one reason you can't help as many people as you would like. Stop living day-to-day and start thinking about the bigger picture of what you're doing. Even the best engines wear out if you don't look after them.

More, if you're always in a bind over a lack of cash, it's easy to overlook the reality of the impact you make on people's lives. It's easy to forget just how much good you're doing. That leads to a loss of positivity in yourself and what your business stands for—and if you're not careful, it's this lack of positivity that wears you down. The struggle in business is real, but it is nearly always self-inflicted.

TELL AN INSURANCE COMPANY TO GO TO HELL

The default mode of most *unconfident* business owners is to keep their rates low and hopefully, eventually, somehow develop the courage and confidence required to raise them. That is how you *could* do it. I'd like to propose we shortcut that process and do it now.

Nothing is stopping you from raising your rates starting today. Nothing except *you*, that is.

Even if you're regulated by some crappy insurance companies, why not drop one of them? Pick the worst-paying one you're contracted to and take great pleasure in sending them a letter with the subject line "Go to hell" or "Stick your crappy $80 reimbursement fees up your ass."

Here's a letter you might want to write them:

"Dear *Soul Sucking* Insurance Company,

Re: Stick your crappy $80 reimbursement fees up your ass

*After years of wondering when the money will flow to me, I've realized that **you're** the reason it isn't. After years of feeling bad about myself, I have at last come to my senses. I've decided that it's time that I moved on and finally start to achieve my full earning potential. With you around, I know that isn't going to happen.*

*Thankfully, I have finally come to the realization that I **am** worth more than the $80 you like to reimburse. From now on, I will be charging your clients $300 per session. They can pay me cash, with a credit card, or via a check. I am not fussy about which one, but it will be upfront at the time of service so that I am never again waiting weeks on end, hoping I didn't mess up the coding.*

From now on, I will be giving your members a level of service that I am proud of; one that makes me feel good about what I do again, and one that makes them feel happy enough to want to keep paying it.

Your measly $80 reimbursements are barely enough to keep the lights on in my clinic and that is why I'd politely like to tell you to stick your reimbursement fees up your ass.

As for your claims department, which always rejected and sent back my bills, I'd like to tell those folks to go to hell. They made my life a misery for years and the only thing that makes me smile is the prospect of one of them having their own claims rejected.

GET YOUR FREE SALES KIT: WWW.PAULGOUGH.COM/SALES-KIT

I would love to end this note by saying that I am going to miss you—but I am not. The only good thing that I can say about our relationship is that it's over.

Thanks for nothing.

Paul "now charging $300 per session" Gough

P.S. *If you need to find another provider of physical therapy to replace me on your low-paid network of providers, please get in touch with me. For an inconvenience fee of $1,000—paid in advance—I will cheerfully provide you with the names and contact details of some of my miserable competitors.*

There are a few physical therapists close by me who I know would love you to suck the life out of them. These therapists are a special breed—they love to work for less than it costs to run their business and for that reason I think you would get on well with each other.

Doing something like this would be worth it just for the uptick in how good you feel about yourself. The next time the phone rings and someone asks if you take their insurance, tell them this: "The good news is we don't." When you do, watch how great you feel inside. Good riddance to the crappy insurance companies and their low reimbursements; they're the primary reason you're struggling to give the level of service you wish you could.

I'll end this section as I started it, with a reminder that charging a low fee for your service is the biggest and most obvious sign that you're not confident in yourself or that you're unsure about what you do and the outcome that you can get for people.

I believe that price is a statement of value: the more you believe you bring, the more you should charge. The more value that they believe you bring, the more they will want to pay. But it starts with you.

GET YOUR FREE SALES KIT: WWW.PAULGOUGH.COM/SALES-KIT

THE "WHEN, THEN" FALLACY

At this point, I know what you're thinking. All of this sounds great, Paul…but I'm just not ready to do it yet. *When* I am a little more experienced or *when* I get some more patients, *then* I will send that letter to the insurance company or raise my rates.

Here's the thing: *"When I get a few more years' experience"* or *"When I get a busy case load,* then *I will raise my rates"* is how most people think. The problem is that is also how they remain.

"When this, then that" is a curse that keeps people stuck.

Thinking that way suggests that something out of your control has to happen before you get the thing you want to control. *When* only ever happens when you make it happen. "When, then" is like the "someday" disease that is slowly killing many people's chances of success.

"Someday I'll get around to raising my rates." No you won't. The reason you couldn't raise your rates ten years ago is *still* the reason you can't raise them today. You're still worried about being judged.

The harsh reality is that most clinic owners never get the patient volume to ever be confident enough to raise their rates. That's because the patients don't want to do business with people who are uncertain about themselves or lack self-confidence. Said differently, it's because your rates are so low that people are being put off from coming. Don't forget that low prices only work to attract patients who are only concerned about price. It only works to attract patients who can't afford to pay for health care and who only want what insurance will cover. It creates a vicious cycle that is virtually impossible to break.

Hard to accept, I know, but it's because your rates are so low that you're stuck in a never-ending loop of having an issue with money and self-worth.

Price is a contentious subject. Price is also a filter. It filters the people looking for certainty and looking for a guaranteed outcome. How you set your prices screams how certain you are in achieving that outcome for them. It does not scream that you're greedy or that you just want to make money. It screams that you're confident and certain in what you do for people. These are the two things people want most, particularly in health care.

I appreciate that there's an issue with money in health care, but I think the only issue you should ever have with money is what to spend it all on. It's a great problem to have—what to do when you get a truckload of cash from running a successful business *that meets the needs of tens of thousands of people who are now living healthier lives.*

Price is simply a product of emotion. There's no real worth to anything. It's not your price that it is ever in question—it is how people feel about it. That is something you can change. Think about it: the price is the price. Some people like it, others question it, some don't blink an eye and others think it's so cheap that there must be a catch. The price hasn't changed and yet everyone has a different opinion on it. This tells you that price is never the issue. The only issue is how they feel about it, and how they are allowed to feel about it is 100 percent in your control.

LEARNING HOW TO CHARGE PROPERLY

Learning how to charge properly is the first step toward affirming to yourself that you are capable of doing what you say you are.

From now on, here's how I want you to position your price to your patients.

When people ask how much you charge, look them straight in the eye and tell them. Whether it is $200 or $300, hit them with it and then hold your composure in the silence that will follow and do nothing but wait for them to respond. Whether they say "yes" or "no," from now on, you don't care.

As I've pointed out a few times already, the key is to not react either way. Be careful not to make any excuses or try to justify your prices. Do not say, "I have to charge you this because of the cost of my rent" or "I have to charge this because I am poor and miserable and having this money might make me happier." Just tell them your fee without any justification and make sure you do it free from guilt.

There's an unbelievable power in telling someone what you want to be paid and then staying silent.

It is irrelevant if they hire you or not. Like I have said before, your feeling of self-worth or importance is not improved by a random person becoming a patient of your clinic. If they say no, *it's their loss*. Never forget that there are tens of thousands of people out there with back pain, but there's only one of you. Start acting like it. This is about you becoming comfortable with telling people that you are worthy of the fee. If you don't think you're worthy, how can you expect them to?

What you charge right now is a reflection of how you feel about yourself. The problem with running a business is that if you're not careful, you feel lousy and insecure most of the time. It is easy to feel like insurance companies, medical doctors and your competitors are conspiring against you. Not to mention that people are more skeptical than ever about paying for health care as the costs continue to rise.

This negativity shows up in your conversations with patients, meaning you've got less energy and less certainty to give them. Because of that, it actually makes charging even low fees more difficult.

It's a hamster wheel that is very easy to get trapped on.

FEEL GOOD, RIGHT NOW

The fastest way to feel better about yourself right now is to raise your rates. It reminds you that you're in control and you're not passively at the mercy of the circus called life that is going on around you.

Before you do it, I know you'll feel sick. Your stomach will churn and you'll shuffle around in your chair to shake off that uncomfortable feeling in your stomach (the one you most likely got as soon as I mentioned you doing it).

This will feel sickening at first, but when you finally do it, it is liberating. The only regret you'll have will be that you didn't do it years ago. You'll also kick yourself when you do the math and realize that if you had done it years ago, you'd have likely paid off your mortgage with the difference in cash you would have made. Or put your kids through college.

Never forget it is okay for you to make some money while simultaneously helping others.

I know this is a radical concept, but I'm in favor of you *serving yourself first for once*. To be constantly serving everyone else is a zero-sum game if you don't protect the person doing the serving. There's a very good reason that the airlines tell you to put on your own oxygen mask before helping someone else. You can't help others if you've passed out. Equally, you're no good to your patients if you're burned out from working every hour just to cover expenses.

You might not like the idea of looking after yourself first, but in order to serve your patients and for your family to be looked after, it is what you absolutely must do.

Charging higher prices is your duty if you want to help people long term. If you're that good at what you do, and I'm one of your patients, I'd rather you charge me more just so that you look after yourself so that you can take care of *me* longer. I'll find the additional money—but if you're that good, I'll never be able to find another one of *you*. If you're burned out, what will I do when I next need my low back or knee looked at?

If you're not around, I'll have to risk going to your crummy competitor who will treat me no better than a billable unit. Please, for my sake as your patient, take care of yourself before anyone else. I *will* thank you for it.

HOW TO ANNOUNCE A RATE INCREASE TO PATIENTS

Hopefully by now you will agree with me that charging higher fees is in everyone's best interest —yours, and your patients'. If we are in agreement, the next thing to do is put it into action. We're going to do it the moment you have finished reading this book. The next time a patient rings up and asks about booking an appointment, I want you to **add $100** to the fee. Gasp!

I've given you a little breathing space there to recover from the shock of reading that last sentence, and to get comfortable again in your seat. Hopefully you're breathing in and out normally again at this point. If you are, we're good to move on.

When the patient asks, "What's the cost?", here's precisely how you're going to respond:

"For your convenience, my fees are now $200."

And then they'll say:

"Hey, but wasn't it only $100 last week? Why is it all of a sudden $200?"

I want you to reply with, "Yes, it was $100 last week, but this week *I feel good about myself* and I intend on making you feel the same. It's $200. Take it or leave it!"

I want you to start seeing yourself as a transfer of energy and certainty. It's been the recurring theme of this book. That's because this is what it takes to sell with ease and integrity. People can get physical therapy anywhere, from anyone. But energy is rare, and certainty is equally as hard to find. When you see yourself as transferring energy in exchange for money, it is much easier to raise rates and charge what you're worth.

There's no particular value to energy, *so there's no limit to what people will pay you.* That's why everything I've outlined to you in this book is what you must do if you want to be free from the shackles of worrying about money or your self-worth.

If you're still not sure, remember that people feel good about themselves when they pay high prices.

When people spend $5,000 on a handbag from Louis Vuitton or $10,000 on a Rolex watch, they don't feel bad because they did—they feel great because they did. Why don't you make your patients feel like they're buying a Bentley instead of a Dodge when they spend money with you?

GET YOUR FREE SALES KIT: WWW.PAULGOUGH.COM/SALES-KIT

As I write this chapter of the book, I've just come from a relaxing spa break at a place close to my home in England. It was chock-full of people happy to be spending money on pampering themselves with things like massages and facials, enjoying a glass of Champagne to boot.

It was ridiculously expensive. Every single treatment was two if not three times the cost of the standard physiotherapy session in the UK, and yet people were paying it in droves. It was also the first week of the new year. Isn't that when they all supposedly have no money to spend?

Well, they didn't appear to be low on money from where I was lying on my lounger and they all looked to be feeling great about spending it too.

The spa we went to is well known for being expensive. *And that is why most people go.* They can't wait to check-in on Facebook, share pictures on Instagram, and let all of their friends know that they're about to pay $100 more for a facial than they could have elsewhere. I spent thirty-six hours in the spa and I didn't see one miserable face, despite the prices. I put it to you that the higher prices made them feel good about themselves.

You might not believe it, but it's 100 percent true. It is happening everywhere. When people pay higher prices, it serves to add to their own self-worth. The fact that they *can* and *are* paying $100 more for their facial gives them a buzz that they wouldn't get if they went to see some lady who does the same treatment in her spare room.

For example: how much buzz do you get out of spending $20 at McDonald's? Very little. By contrast, how about a $300 meal at Morton's The Steakhouse? Now that makes you feel special, right? You have to spend more money in quality places, but you also get more for doing so. People usually want more for their money and they've proven that they're happy to do so.

CHEAP ATTRACTS CHEAP

The point of that story? I assume that you believe that you're a quality place for people to spend their money. If you do, give it to them by charging them for it. Just bill them for it when they show up.

What is more, the more you charge, the more they respect you. I've yet to have been in a Morton's or Fleming's restaurant and observe the staff take hassle or flak from the customers. However, in McDonald's, it's rare that I'll even hear a "please" or "thank you" from the customer or the staff. I never leave McDonald's feeling ecstatic about myself or my purchase and that's because it is cheap.

If you do things on the cheap, people tend to get down on you and find fault with what you do. Having gotten something for nothing, they begin to demand even more. In all of my businesses, it's always the ones that pay the least who give me the most hassle.

The other emotion about charging higher prices is fear of loss. We tend to feel that if we charge a large amount, somehow all of our patients will disappear and we'll have to close the clinic by Wednesday next week.

Yet, despite recession after recession, more skepticism and fearmongering by the media than ever before, quality items continue to be bought and sold. Expensive items like Bentleys, French Champagne, and five-star hotels all *still* exist during and after a recession and they usually do better in bad times. Why? It's because in bad times people want to feel good about themselves. They do that by shopping with people who they know will help them to achieve that state.

Which companies struggle during the bad times? It's the companies that charge "average" prices or are somewhere in the middle. Even the dollar stores are starting to go bust.

To make this work for you, all you have to do is agree that what you do is quality—and charge appropriately for it.

It's easy to look at all of your competitors and feel restricted by charging more. It's tempting to look at your competition who have possibly been in business longer than you and assume that because you're new or smaller, you can never possibly beat them or charge a higher price.

Well, if you compete on providing physical therapy, you never will. But if you do any of even just some of what I've outlined in this book, you will be more than okay.

GET YOUR FREE SALES KIT: WWW.PAULGOUGH.COM/SALES-KIT

YOUR BORING COMPETITORS

For the most part, all of your competitors are the same. Their websites look the same, the way they answer the phone is the same (dull and boring), their clinics look the same (with dull and boring colors on the wall), their marketing is the same (lame) and their prices are the same—too low. It means their results are the same: *very little profit for a lot of hassle and a whole bunch of heartache.*

It's worth it for people to pay an extra $50 to not have to go through the hassle and emotion of hiring a "regular" service and not getting what they wanted.

Heck, I'd pay $50 more just to have the phone answered the first time I ring most healthcare clinics and have one of them remember my first name when I walk in.

This game of business is really not that difficult to win: just give people what they really want and when you do, *bill them for it* appropriately knowing that in doing so you can continue to do it for them any time their need arises. *Bill them for it* appropriately knowing you can provide the level of service that makes them feel good about themselves because they did business with you.

In a world where most everything is ordinary, where things are churned out the same way year after year, it is not that difficult to get ahead and have people thrilled about paying more to hire you. If you come from a place of originality, invest energy in things, and hire people with energy who project certainty, then people will respond.

It all starts by charging at a level that means you can provide a level of service that people actually want to pay for. Choose your prices wisely. The future of your business really does depend upon it.

GET YOUR FREE SALES KIT: WWW.PAULGOUGH.COM/SALES-KIT

TALK TO ME AS YOU MOVE THROUGH THE BOOK:

LET ME KNOW YOUR THOUGHTS AND COMMENTS OVER ON TWITTER OR INSTAGRAM:

@THEPAULGOUGH // #ASKPG

GET YOUR FREE SALES KIT: WWW.PAULGOUGH.COM/SALES-KIT

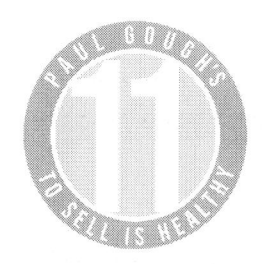

GET THE COMPLETE SALES AND CONVERSION SYSTEM FOR PHYSICAL THERAPISTS

If you're still reading at this point, hopefully you'll agree with me that it is okay to sell in health care. Ideally, you now believe it is neither good nor bad—it is much needed. Much like a massage or a set of exercises, selling is a tool that exists for the purpose of helping someone live a more active and healthy life.

Far from being something that is being done *to them*, it is a skill you will develop that will ultimately affect their life positively. It is a service that they don't know how to ask for, yet when they experience it, it will leave them feeling that there was something easy and effortless about the way in which they came to the decision to hire you.

Sure, there will be one or two people who don't like the idea of someone being *supremely confident* enough to stand up and sell what they do with poise and integrity—but don't let that person spoil it for the hundreds of others whose *lives you will change* by simply changing your own view of selling.

If you do get the odd one or two people not happy with your newfound level of certainty and confidence in yourself, simply do as I do and send them to your competitors.

I have a list of all my competitor's phone numbers on each reception desk and my front desk team is instructed to direct anyone who doesn't like my approach to one of them, with my compliments. I think the line we use is, "If you tell them Paul Gough sent you, you might get a discount on their already cheap service."

If nothing else, it brightens my day to know that my competitor is having to explain why they can't give them a discount because they know Paul Gough.

GET YOUR FREE SALES KIT: WWW.PAULGOUGH.COM/SALES-KIT

If ever you're a little uneasy in selling or raising prices, the thing that you should ask yourself is, "What's my intent?" The answer to that question ends all of the conflict.

I assume that, like me, your intent is to help someone live a more active and healthy life? To give them something that will enhance their life? Remember that you're not knocking on doors, mercilessly trying to sell things to people who don't have the problems your service solves. No, it's quite the reverse. You and I are selling a vital solution that transforms people's lives and we're only doing it for people who have told us that they're suffering.

They're knocking on *our* doors asking about *our* solution.

As I like to put it, you have their transformation and they have your money. Don't let a lack of confidence or a false belief about money get in the way of an exchange taking place.

Asking yourself, "What is my intent?" is a great way of giving yourself the immediate confidence to carry through with what I've taught you in the pages of this book and *influence with integrity*. In doing so, you will help significantly more people live active and healthy lives than you are right now.

WHAT ARE YOU REALLY SELLING?

With that in mind, I'd like to close this book with a reminder of what you're really selling people as a physical therapist. It's very easy to think that because you're a physical therapist, what you sell is physical therapy. But that's just *how* you do what you really do. What you're really selling people is *certainty, hope, a memorable experience, and a transformation* in someone's health. These are the things that people *really* want. Let's take a closer look at how important each one is.

CERTAINTY

The only thing worse than being in pain is being indecisive over what to do about that pain. There's very little progress in life when someone is uncertain. Your job is to make them feel certain in themselves and in you, to sell them on that feeling. When a patient feels certain, they also feel safe. If they feel safe, they'll start to make their way toward the solution that they need. That's you.

Being absolutely certain in your ability to help them—even if it is only by getting them 20 to 30 percent better than they are now—is the best way to make someone feel instantly better about themselves and what is possible for their future. You have the ability to make them feel certain in themselves again—sell it to them and they'll buy your physical therapy skills.

HOPE

When you're in pain or suffering, it's not long before you start to wonder if the thing you've got will ever go away. Most of your patients have suffered for so long already. They have tried so many things that have so far not worked that they've almost *given up hope* of ever being able to wake up and not have pain in their knee or back. You have the ability to give them this hope back. Sell it to them—and they'll buy your physical therapy skills at twice the price.

A MEMORABLE EXPERIENCE

Most places that your patients go, they are getting a dreadful experience. They're talking to people who hate their jobs, hate their lives, and are so mind-numbingly bored that they're literally sleepwalking their way through their days. And that's me being polite.

Commit to doing whatever it takes to being the standout interaction they have with anyone vying for their business. Commit to brightening their day so that you make them feel much better about themselves emotionally, not just physically. They'll always pay you more for massaging their ego than their hamstring.

It can be as simple as having your front desk person remembering their name and actually using it when they walk in. In doing so, you're elevating your patients to a feeling of being recognized. That feeling is usually reserved for celebrities. They'll pay you for that.

GET YOUR FREE SALES KIT: WWW.PAULGOUGH.COM/SALES-KIT

It could be as "fancy" as ensuring their favorite cup of coffee is ready for them—before they get into the clinic. Why should they have to ask, anyway? After all, they've had the same cup of coffee, made the same way, the last four times they've been in. Don't ask them a fifth time what they want. You already know. It'll make the coffee taste much nicer to know that you noticed what they want and acted on it.

People will always forget what you did, but they'll always remember how you made them feel. Sell that to them—and they'll buy your physical therapy services at twice the price.

A TRANSFORMATION

You're not just fixing knee pain; you are literally transforming their health. You're giving them the ability to walk along the beach with their husband or wife and enjoy watching the beautiful sunset. You're giving them the ability to sleep at night and get more living out of the next day. You're keeping them active and mobile with a better chance of avoiding dangerous surgery. You're giving them their independence and ensuring their self-worth is preserved for years longer than it might have been.

You're transforming their life by restoring their health—sell it to them and they'll buy your physical therapy services at twice the price.

Like I said at the very start of this book, getting better at selling *physical therapy* is not the answer. The only solution to selling more and increasing your prices is to sell something entirely different from everyone else. Do it right, and the process of selling becomes **EFFORTLESS**. It's why I call successful selling "Effortless Selling" and created an entire system around it.

If you're continuously being price shopped, sell them something that cannot be price shopped. All of the things I've just described are impossible for anyone to put a comparable price on.

I can't ever imagine a patient ringing up and asking your competitors how much they charge for *renewed hope, a celebrity-like experience, and absolute certainty that culminates in a total health transformation.* Can you?

On the contrary, your patients can easily assign what they believe to be a fair price to McKenzie exercises or your dry needling services. With a mobile phone in their hands and Google at the ready, they can do that simply by calling around to three of your competitors.

WHAT'S IN IT FOR YOU—A NEW YACHT?

If the patient gets the reward of *certainty, hope, an unforgettable experience, and a total transformation in their health*, then what's in it for you? If you're doing all of this for them, what do you get in return? For this to work and to be sustained, you have to get something out of it too. There's nothing on Earth that can sustain giving without receiving something in return.

I believe the greatest gift you will ever get from doing all of this *for* people is an unrivaled level of fulfillment. That is to live with the satisfaction of knowing that you've given all that you've got and done all that you know to enhance someone else's life.

There may be more that can be done, but fulfillment is knowing that you've done all that you currently know. You went onto the field and left nothing in the locker room, so to speak.

Of course, the additional cash is very nice, too. With more of it, you can go off and do things that you otherwise wouldn't have been able to do or experience.

Anyone who says that money doesn't make you happy has never had any. Believe me, I'm way happier when I'm flying first class across the Atlantic Ocean for nine hours than if I'm crammed in the middle seat in economy.

Best, when you're living a life that is fulfilled and you're free from the pressure cooker that having no cash creates, you bring even more value to the lives of the people you're serving.

Agree or disagree, cash *is* the gateway to you having more time to think about how you can better serve people.

Instead of worrying about how you're going to pay your credit card bills, you're thinking of ways to improve your service or add more benefits to your practice. You're living in a world of abundance instead of drought. You're thinking about what else you can *give* instead of what you have to *give up*.

That has surely got to be the type of life you want. That has to be the life *everyone* should want. To do anything otherwise is to think that you don't deserve to be fulfilled or that it is somehow wrong to be rich.

Next time you see someone really rich, commit to being happy for them. If you do, you're agreeing that it is possible and that it is okay. If you see someone really rich and you have negative thoughts about them—just for being rich—then you're telling yourself it is wrong even though there's no grounds for thinking that way.

It's only the government that punishes you for being rich, and they're only doing so to make up for all the mistakes they keep making with everyone's money. Is it a trillion dollars of debt, or two?

Some politicians might want to give everyone everything for free—and a lot of people applaud them when it is suggested—but how is it all paid for? That's right, it's the people with money who are taxed. Making a lot more cash means you have helped a lot of people. That is positive capitalism at its best. Call me old fashioned, but I still believe in a world where if you do something good, and you work to create more value than anyone else, then you absolutely should get rewarded with the money needed to do the things in your life that *make being in business worthwhile*.

What I am trying to say is never feel bad or guilty about having money. It is simply a reward that the world recognizes as being significant. Money is the only way people know how to compensate you for your value. If they want to compensate you with money, why waste energy resisting it? Smile, say "thank you" as you accept it—and then spend it wisely.

I love Warren Buffett's take on money. He sees it as a measure of the number of good decisions that have been made in his business. Meaning, the more money that is in the bank, the more good decisions have been made. It doesn't mean anything good, or anything bad, it just means that someone made some good decisions and, because of the way the world works, more money flowed in his direction.

GET YOUR FREE SALES KIT: WWW.PAULGOUGH.COM/SALES-KIT

You and I are not capable of reprogramming the way the world works when it comes to compensating good work with money. It's ignorant to think we are. The only thing you can do is agree to get in the way of where it flows so that more of it makes its way to you. When you get it, do as you please. Give it to charity, give it to your kids, stockpile it and sit on it and look at it every day if that floats your boat.

BUY YOURSELF A NEW YACHT

Speaking of boats, if you want to treat yourself to a new yacht, go get one. And don't worry for one second about what your staff or patients will think. Tell them they can come on board with you any time they like. Better yet, let them take their family out on it so they can get a whiff of what it feels like to *have helped so many people so profoundly*. If anyone questions your new yacht, remind them that the money available to you is directly proportional to the amount of *certainty, hope, and health transformations* that you have provided for people.

Imagine being a multimillionaire private practice owner and saying that you achieved real wealth because you transformed ten thousand people's lives. That has to be better than being yet another struggling physical therapist, spending your whole life blaming your money issues on insurance companies or on the issues your family had three generations ago.

I appreciate that some people are addicted to the struggle. But I sincerely believe that the best thing you can do for struggling clinic owners is agree *not to join them*. Refuse to take part in their *self-pity party*.

It is the same with people who are struggling or poor in life. The best way to help them is to make a commitment to not join them. Help them up by showing them what is possible when you decide to take control of your own life, your own decisions, and your own actions. Including how much money you want to make and what you want to spend it on.

I guess what I am saying is how this all ends is up to you. How it will look at the end of your private practice career is up to you. You can be another run-of-the-mill clinic owner who only just scraped by, or you can make a massive impact on people and you can *all* enjoy the fact that you did.

I don't know how much impact or how much profit you will make, but what I do know is that to do either of those things you're going to have to *sell to people* and *you're going to have to charge appropriately for it*. Whether you have a mattress stuffed with cash because you made so much of it you that couldn't find a bank to store it all or you wind up struggling to pay the mortgage off and have to work at McDonald's just to get health insurance, it is your choice.

If you've started a private practice, then you're in a privileged position to determine your own destiny, and I believe that is a privilege that you must exercise. For all of the reasons we've discussed in this book, you owe it to yourself, your family, and your patients to make the most of everything you've got—cash included.

ADD $77,000 IN PROFIT DOING JUST THESE THREE THINGS

Just before we close out the book, I'd like to show how close you are to making a bigger impact—and therefore making a lot more money—at your practice. I want to share with you my formula for calculating your clinic's **Profitability Potential**. Wherever you are starting from, it's likely that you're just one or two steps away from adding an additional $77,000 to your bottom line.

I appreciate that making an extra $77,000 seems like it could take you a lot of time or require a lot of work. But that isn't true. When it comes to improving your profit, improving sales is the fastest and easiest way to do it. Unlike any other way to grow a business, improving your sales doesn't come with any additional expense. You have to pay the rent, staff, and insurance regardless. That is why you should make improving your clinic's sales and conversion system your number one priority when you put down this book.

Even if you're getting just one person you currently can't convert, there's a lot of money sitting there waiting for you to claim it.

The path to an extra $77,000 is to get **just one** extra patient each week that you're currently losing (because you can't convert), who will spend an extra $50 with you each time, and have that same person take an extra three sessions with you.

Here's how it works:

Step 1. Get just one additional patient to say "yes" to you each week. If your patient averages five sessions in a plan of care and you charge $150 per session, with that one additional conversion you just added $750 per week ($35,000 extra per year).

Step 2. Next, raise your rates by $50. That brings in an extra $250 per patient. Meaning, you've added another $12,000 per year in additional sales from that one extra conversion per week.

Step 3. Finally, confidently recommend the eight sessions they need to have their health *transformed* (instead of settling on five sessions that will only ease pain). That will bring in an additional $600 per converted patient at your new rate of $200 per session. That brings in another $30,000 per year.

In total, doing just those three things has added $77,000 to your profit—and that is with just one extra patient that you otherwise would have lost.

If you get two extra patients, it will be double that amount. If you get three (easily doable), it would be more than $200,000.

I mean it when I say I don't think clinic owners realize just how close they are to taking home an additional **$100,000 in profit**. It's not about how much you work or how hard you work—it's always about *what* you're working on and that should be your sales

YOUR OPPORTUNITY TO STUDY WITH PAUL AFTER THIS BOOK

As you can see, there's nothing more impactful to work on than your clinic's sales and conversion system. It is one of the highest-value activities you will ever do.

Would you like some more help from me to optimize your system so that we can make that profit potential a reality?

GET YOUR FREE SALES KIT: WWW.PAULGOUGH.COM/SALES-KIT

It was my full intention to use the pages of this book to make you aware of what is required to confidently sell your services at significantly higher prices. This book was about showing you that there absolutely is a way to sell in health care without being salesy. What is more, I wanted you to know that yes, it absolutely is okay to sell your services at higher prices, free from guilt or worrying over what others think of you. Finally, and most importantly, I wanted you to see that you are right to want to make as much money as you can from your business for you and your family's sake.

This book was the *first step* on your journey to building a sales and conversion system that will double, triple, and quadruple your clinic profits. Having an effective sales and conversion system is likely to be the final missing link between making all of the money you want or continuing to struggle along for years to come. Now that you've successfully completed the first step, there's a couple more that I invite you to take with me so that we can build a world-class sales and conversion system at your clinic.

OPTION 1: FREE SALES TRAINING WEBINAR

In this free online training, I revisit many of the principles I outlined in this book. If you want to hear me speak about the principles behind successful selling in a little more depth, then I recommend you do that next. The title of the free webinar is, "How to Sell Physical Therapy—Without Being 'Salesy'."

YOU'LL DISCOVER:

- How to increase your sales by 100 percent by doing just three things

- How to raise cash rates above $250 (without getting pushback or losing patients)

- The priming effect—what it is and how to use it to answer the "Do you take my insurance?" question

GET YOUR FREE SALES KIT: WWW.PAULGOUGH.COM/SALES-KIT

- The seven common objections to cash pay physical therapy and high copays (and why each one really happens)

- The five essential steps of any profitable physical therapy sales system

- Three questions to ask to get a completed plan of care more frequently

- How to overcome the fear of selling

JOIN THE FREE TRAINING HERE:
WWW.PAULGOUGH.COM/SALES-TRAINING

OPTION 2: GET THE COMPLETE "EFFORTLESS SELLING SYSTEM"

Get the Complete "Effortless Selling System: Double Your Front Desk and Treatment Room Conversions in Just 48 hours" - Instant Access 8 Module Program (with all the scripts and training videos you'll need to convert more patients at much higher prices).

This is where we put all of this talk about making more profit into *action!* Get all the resources, scripts, and blueprints that you need to overcome any objection, convert more patients on the phone, and get more people to complete a full plan of care—at twice the price you are charging now. This is everything you need to create a stunningly successful sales and conversion system that will add tens of thousands of extra dollars *per month* to your profit.

THIS INSTANT ACCESS PROGRAM IS FOR YOU IF:

- You've read the book and now you want the exact scripts and templates to finally sort out your conversion issues

- You've read the book and you've decided you're done with charging such low rates

- You're getting inquires, but you're hearing "I'll have to think about it" more times than you would like

- Patients often tell you they want to use their insurance first—and you don't feel comfortable with challenging that objection

- Patients are regularly telling you that the copay cost is an issue—but you don't know how to overcome it or what to say in response

- Your marketing is working well and you're getting enough new leads, but you can't get them on the schedule

- Patients tell you they only want a couple of sessions and not the full plan of care you recommend

- Patients are telling you they can't come more than once per week because their copay or deductible is so high—even though you know they need to

- You don't know how to justify being a cash pay physical therapist

- When you do get inquiries from Google, Facebook, or your website, not enough are converting to paying patients

- You've heard that many cash physical therapists are charging far more than $250 per session and you're finally ready to join them

DETAILS HERE:
WWW.PATIENTCONVERSIONSYSTEM.COM/BOOK

When you get your hands on the instant access program, you will be able to master *all* of the scenarios that require you to sell, including:

1. Converting "cold leads" (from your website, Google, Facebook, etc.) to full paying patients

2. Selling value on the phone to "warm leads" (those folks who requested your free reports or made inquires about price)

GET YOUR FREE SALES KIT: WWW.PAULGOUGH.COM/SALES-KIT

3. Converting people at the initial consultation (to a full plan of care)

4. Converting from discovery visits/taster sessions

5. Reselling the value of physical therapy to patients who have dropped off or did not show

6. Selling and converting at in-clinic workshops or when speaking at educational events

When you enroll in the "Effortless Selling System" program you are getting instant access to everything you need to create a sales and conversion system that make objections a thing or the past, including scripts for your staff!

HERE ARE SOME OF THE LESSONS:

Lesson 1: The Fundamentals of Sales—PLUS, 14 Simple Ways to Optimize Your Conversion System

Lesson 2: Influence & The Five Levels of Persuasive Communication

Lesson 3: Essential Sales Strategies Perfect For Health Care Providers

Lesson 4: Selling To Serve

Lesson 5: Overcoming the Seven Most Common Objections to Paying Cash for Physical Therapy (Precisely What To Say)

Lesson 6: Front Desk Phone Sales: How To Get Them Off The Phone And Into Your Clinic

Lesson 7: Treatment Room Conversions: How To Convert To A Full Plan Of Care

Lesson 8: Maximizing Sales: Raising Rates, Cash Up-Sells and Re-Activating Drop-Offs

GET YOUR FREE SALES KIT: WWW.PAULGOUGH.COM/SALES-KIT

GET MY "SAY THIS, SAY THAT" PHONE AND IN-CLINIC SCRIPTS

Plus, you'll be able to download all the slides with the exact words, scripts, and verbiage you need to custom tailor the perfect sales conversion for your type of practice.

DETAILS HERE:
WWW.PATIENTCONVERSIONSYSTEM.COM/BOOK

SAVE $500 USING THIS COUPON CODE

Use This Coupon Code To Save
An Additional $500 While the Coupon Lasts

BOOK500

FREE BONUS: TWO TICKETS TO MY LIVE
SALES AND CONVERSION 2-DAY BOOTCAMP

Plus, when you order the instant access Effortless Selling System program, you'll also get two free tickets to my annual 2-Day Sales and Conversion Bootcamp.

At this live bootcamp, you will work with me personally and I can ensure you get the absolute best ROI on your new sales and conversion system. When you implement everything, you'll discover in the online program, you're ready to work with me in person and we can take your profits to new heights.

You've read the book, the best thing to do next is to take the instant access training and then come and perfect your sales and conversion system with me in person at the next bootcamp.

When you order the online program, simply reply to the confirmation email and ask for details on the next live two-day training. We'll be in touch to let you know when it is and give you all the details.

DETAILS HERE:
WWW.PATIENTCONVERSIONSYSTEM.COM/BOOK

To your success,

Paul Gough

P.S Here's what people have to say about how they've been impacted since taking this remarkable "Effortless Selling System" program:

"Before Paul's Effortless Selling program I used to dread the phone ringing – I was always worried about hearing the words most Cash PT's dread, "do you take my insurance…" Now all of that has changed. This program has taken my confidence to the next level. I'm now equipped with a clear framework to handle objections, I don't feel like I'm winging it, desperately trying to convince someone to pay for my services, and even better - my staff have the skills to confidently convert inquires to actual paying patients and at more than $100."
Carrie Jose Gove, CJ Physical Therapy, Portsmouth, NH

"How was I able to convert over $6000 worth of new patients in my first month of business? It was because of everything I learned from Paul Gough and specifically his Effortless Selling System. I learned how to raise rates and how to overcome objections. Without this program I would never of had the skills to convert even half of my leads, not to mention my rates would be a fraction of what they are now."
Joshua Hall, Hall Physical Therapy, Salt Lake City, Utah

GET YOUR FREE SALES KIT: WWW.PAULGOUGH.COM/SALES-KIT

ABOUT THE AUTHOR:

PAUL GOUGH is the No.1 bestselling author of "The New Patient Accelerator Method", and "The Physical Therapy Hiring Solution", two revolutionary books on marketing and hiring for physical therapists. He's also an international speaker and a former professional soccer physical therapist turned successful clinic owner from the UK. Paul is the founder of the Paul Gough Physio Rooms – a successful four location cash pay clinic that he started from a spare room in his home whilst having had no money and no business or marketing skills. Paul has since scaled his clinic from a zero to $1m +, and what's most impressive is that he's done all of that in a country with a completely free, "socialist" health care system (one that provides physical therapy services for FREE for all UK residents) as his main competitor.

He is a true small business success story; he is now the owner of five companies, all of which are in three different markets and in two different countries – two of those companies have achieved million dollar+ revenues.

Paul is the host of the top-rated podcast "The Paul Gough Audio Experience: Business Lessons For Physical Therapists" (available on iTunes, Soundcloud, Spotify, Anchor and Stitcher). He is also a "Small Business ICON" WINNER of the Infusionsoft award for "best in class lead nurture marketing" in 2016, an award that is selected from all across Infusionsoft's 45,000+ global customers.

He is widely regarded, both in America and around the world, as a leading authority on direct to consumer marketing, and he has a proven track record of helping physical therapists attract cash pay patients, growing their practices, increasing profits, freeing up their time, and radically shifting their entrepreneurial thinking. Every week, 10,000's of physical therapists receive his support/advice online and attend his seminars. His business success coaching programs are almost always full.

BE SURE TO CONNECT WITH PAUL ON SOCIAL MEDIA AND LET HIM KNOW HOW THIS BOOK MADE AN IMPACT ON YOU OVER ON TWITTER OR INSTAGRAM: @THEPAULGOUGH, #ASKPG

GET YOUR FREE SALES KIT: WWW.PAULGOUGH.COM/SALES-KIT

OTHER BOOKS IN THE SERIES:

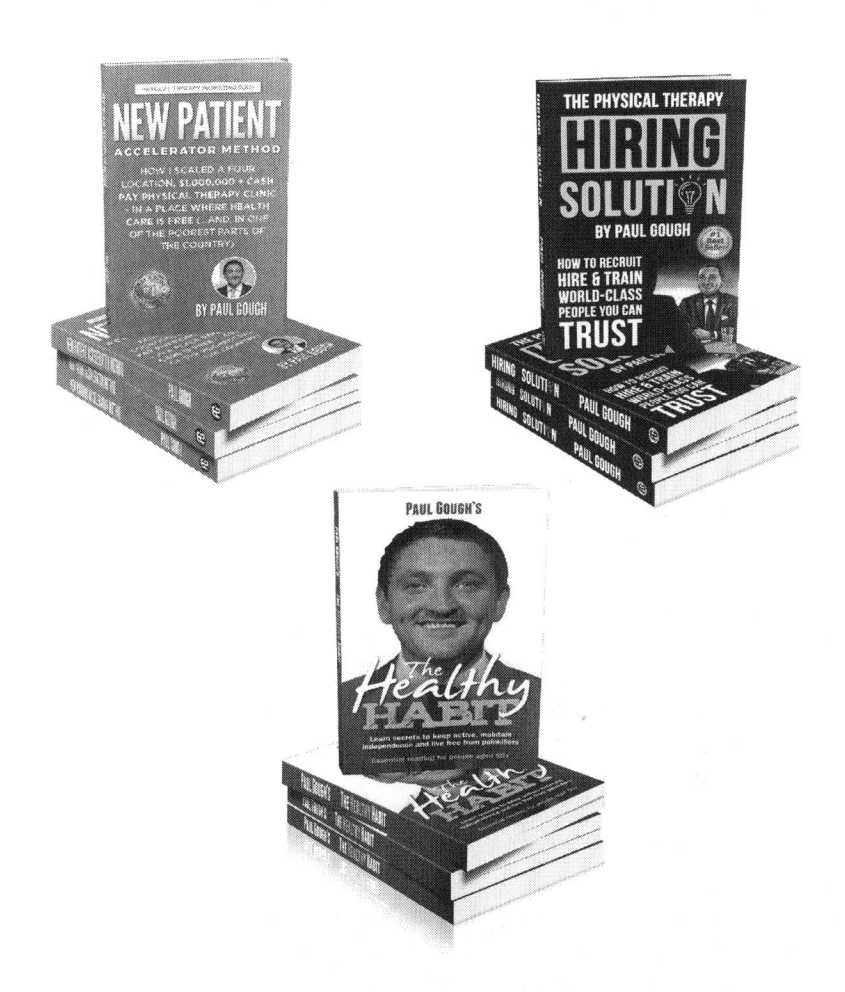

New Patient Accelerator Method:
www.PaulsMarketingBook.com

The Physical Therapy Hiring Solution:
www.PaulsHiringBook.com

The Healthy Habit:
www.PaulsHealthyHabit.com

GET YOUR FREE SALES KIT: WWW.PAULGOUGH.COM/SALES-KIT

164 @THEPAULGOUGH

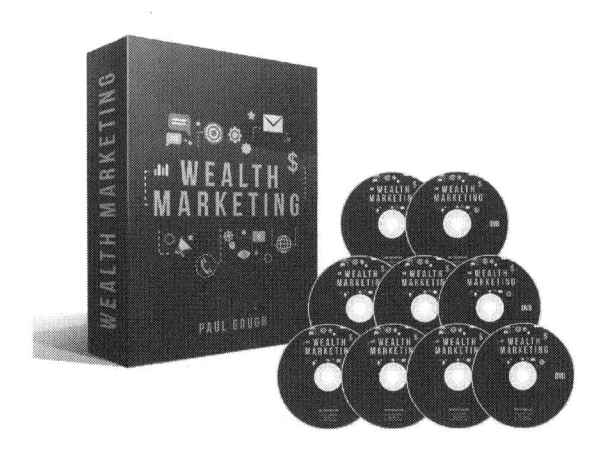

GET YOUR FREE WEALTH MARKETING GIFT FROM PAUL, NOW...

Go to: www.paulgough.com/wealth-gift
To get this instant access 9 DVD video program, NOW.

Claim your $1,997.00 worth of cash patient generating, higher profit making, wealth marketing DVD program, absolutely FREE!

Including a FREE "Test-Drive" of Paul Gough's Cash Club Membership that sends to your clinic $10,000 worth of marketing ideas every 30 days.

Claim your copy now, at
www.paulgough.com/wealth-gift

GET YOUR FREE SALES KIT: WWW.PAULGOUGH.COM/SALES-KIT

Made in the USA
Monee, IL
11 April 2023